Nothing About Us Without Us

NOTHING ABOUT US WITHOUT US

Disability Oppression and Empowerment

James I. Charlton

UNIVERSITY OF CALIFORNIA PRESS

Berkeley / Los Angeles / London

University of California Press
Berkeley and Los Angeles, California

University of California Press
London, England

Library of Congress Cataloging-in-Publication Data

Charlton, James I.
    Nothing about us without us : disability oppression and
empowerment / James I. Charlton.
        p.   cm.
    Includes bibliographical references and index.
    ISBN 0-520-20795-5 (alk. paper)
    1. Handicapped—Civil rights. 2. Handicapped—Social conditions.
    3. Discrimination against the handicapped. 4. Sociology of
disability. 5. Stigma (Social psychology) I. Title.
HV1568.C37 1998
323.3'087—DC21   97-1661
                                                        CIP

Printed in the United States of America

1 2 3 4 5 6 7 8 9

The paper used in this publication meets the minimum requirements of American National Standard for Information Sciences—Permanence of Paper for Printed Library Materials, ANSI Z39.49-1984⊖

To My Mother and Father for Everything

*To Ed Roberts and the Movement
He Touched*

Contents

viii   CONTENTS

The Argument

The lived oppression that people with disabilities have experienced and continue to experience is a human rights tragedy of epic proportions. Only in the last few decades has this begun to be recognized and resisted. Today, in fact, we are witnessing a profound sea change among people with disabilities. For the first time, a movement of people with disabilities has emerged in every region of the world which is demanding a recognition of their human rights and their central role in determining those rights.

There are a number of unifying arguments that run throughout this book which attempt to synthesize both the conditions of disability oppression and the exigencies of its resistance: (1) the oppression of 500 million people with disabilities is rooted in the political-economic and cultural dimensions of everyday life; (2) the poverty, isolation, indignity, and dependence of these 500 million people with disabilities is evidence of a major human rights catastrophe and a fundamental critique of the existing world system; (3) the scant attempts to theorize the conditions of everyday life for people with disabilities are either incomplete or fundamentally flawed as a result of the medicalization/depoliticization of disability and the failure to account for the vast majority of people with disabilities who live in the Third World; (4) a disability-based consciousness and organization is emerging throughout the world which has begun to contest both the oppression people with disabilities experience and the depoliticization of that experience; (5) the political-economic and sociocultural dimensions of disability oppression determine who is

affected and the form resistance takes; (6) notwithstanding the importance of political-economic and sociocultural differences, all the individuals and organizations that have taken up the cause of disability rights in
the last twenty years have embraced the concepts of empowerment and
human rights, independence and integration, and self-help and self-
determination; and (7) these leitmotifs suggest a necessarily fundamental reordering of global priorities and resources based on equality, respect,
and control of resources by the people and communities that need them.

Acknowledgments

I have been thinking about the subject matter of this book since 1985 when I met people associated with the Organización de Revolucionarios Deshabilidades (ORD) in Managua, Nicaragua. It was in the midst of the proxy war the United States was waging against that country, and although the devastation was widespread, it was quickly evident that ORD had been responsible for many impressive changes for people like myself in their country.

By then I had been to Latin America many times, but I had not previously met other politically active people with disabilities. My experience in Nicaragua motivated me to seek out similar experiences elsewhere. In 1991 I received funding from the Institute on Disability at the University of New Hampshire. This grant allowed me to spend a month with members of the National Council of Disabled Persons Zimbabwe (NCDPZ), an extraordinary disability rights organization. In 1992 I received a one-year fellowship from the Chicago Community Trust, and it is with their assistance that most of the research for this book was done. During that year I visited Mexico, Brazil, South Africa, Kenya, India, Thailand, Indonesia, and Hong Kong.

Much of the credit for the insights in this book goes to my colleagues in the disability rights movement in the United States, especially my comrades in Chicago. I am also indebted to dear friends with whom I have been engaged in political projects over the last twenty-five years. I would like to thank Access Living of Metropolitan Chicago, where I have worked since 1985, for providing me with love, encouragement, and sensibility. I would also like to acknowledge the contacts provided me by the World Institute on Disability in Oakland and Disabled Peoples' International in Winnipeg.

Those who assisted me with ideas, comments, and contacts are too numerous to mention here, but I must single out a few of them: Caroline Harney, Tom Wilson, James Potter, Nancy Reed, Roberto Rey, Alexander Phiri, Rebecca Gonzales, Mauricio Ortiz, Orlando Perez, Friday Mavuso, Marceo Oliviero, Ed Roberts, Marca Bristo, Rosangela Berman, Diane Woods, Susan Nussbaum, Terry Turner, and Mel Rothenberg. I will always be grateful for the support of Stan Holwitz and Michelle Nordon and the editorial suggestions of Sheila Berg at the University of California Press.

People Interviewed

I have had the good fortune to interview disability rights activists over the course of many years in the following countries: the United States, Mexico (numerous trips, 1984–1995), Nicaragua (1985), Cuba (1989), Brazil (1988, 1992), Zimbabwe (1991), South Africa (1992), India (1993), Thailand (1993), Indonesia (1993), Hong Kong (1993), and England and Sweden (1995–1996).

The following people are the disability rights activists interviewed. I have provided the organizational affiliation they had at the time of the interview when useful. I do so for identification purposes only as each individual was expressing his or her own political analysis unless otherwise indicated.

The Americas

Felipe Barrera, disabled combatant, activist, San Salvador, El Salvador

Rosangela Berman Bieler, president, Centro de Vida Independente do Rio de Janeiro (CVI, Center for Independent Living), Rio de Janeiro, Brazil

Gabriella Brimmer, poet, member, Asociación de Personas con Impedimentos Fisicos (Association of Persons with Physical Impediments); Asociación para los Derechos de Persons con Alteraciones

Motoras (ADEPAM, Association for the Rights of Persons with Different Mobility), Mexico City

Maria Luiza Camêra, writer, activist, Salvador, Brazil

Angel Pla Cisneros, economic development secretary, Asociación Cubana de Limitados Fisicos Motores (Association of Cubans with Physical Motor Limitations, ACLIFIM), Havana, Cuba

Maria da Comceição Caussat, attorney, activist, Rio de Janeiro, Brazil

Mike Ervin, local coordinator, ADAPT, Chicago, Illinois

Ida Hilda Escalona del Toro, presidente, ACLIFIM, Havana, Cuba

Paulo Saturnino Figueiredo, activist, Belo Horizonte, Brazil

Federico Fleischmann, president, Libre Acceso, A.C. (Free Access), Mexico City

Arnaldo Godoy, city council member, activist, Belo Horizonte, Brazil

Pablo Medina, military commandant, Sandinista Front; member of Organización de Revolucionarios Deshabilitados (Organization of Disabled Revolutionaries, ORD), León, Nicaragua

Cornelio Nuñez Ordaz, president, Asociación Oaxaqueña de Desportes sobres Silla de Reuda, A.C. (Wheelchair Sports Association of Oaxaca), Oaxaca, Mexico

Orlando Perez, external secretary, ORD, Managua, Nicaragua

Judy Panko Reis, administrative director, Health Clinic for Women with Disabilities, Chicago, Illinois

Ed Roberts, president, World Institute on Disability, Oakland, California

Fernando Rodriguez, founder, Mobility International chapter, Mexico City

Jose Luis Silva Trujillo, vice president, ACLIFIM, Havana, Cuba

Maria Paula Teperino, attorney, board member CVI, Rio de Janeiro, Brazil

Freddie Trejos, founder, ORD, Managua, Nicaragua

Nancy Ward, national coordinator, People First, Lincoln, Nebraska

Southern Africa

Susan Berde, member, volunteer, National Council for the Deaf, Johannesburg, South Africa

Fadila Lagadien, member, Disabled People South Africa (DPSA), editor *disABILITY* (DPSA newsletter), Cape Town, South Africa

Joshua Malinga, chairperson, Disabled Peoples' International (DPI); general secretary, Southern Africa Federation of the Disabled (SAFOD); mayor, Bulawayo, Zimbabwe

Lizzie Mamvura, women's coordinator, National Council of Disabled Persons of Zimbabwe (NCDPZ), Bulawayo, Zimbabwe

Michael Masutha, director of socioeconomic rights, Lawyers for Human Rights, member, DPSA, Johannesburg, South Africa

Friday Mandla Mavuso, chairperson and manager, Self-Help Association of Paraplegics (SHAP), Soweto; co-chairperson, economic development, DPSA, Booysens, South Africa

Rangarirai Mupindu, executive director, NCDPZ, Bulawayo, Zimbabwe

Alexander Phiri, chairperson, NCDPZ, Bulawayo, Zimbabwe

William Rowland, general secretary, DPSA, Pretoria, South Africa

Asia

Panomwan Bootem, president, National Association of the Deaf in Thailand, Bangkok

Peter F. S. Chan, chairperson, Rehabilitation Alliance Hong Kong, Kowloon

Danilo B. Delfin, regional development officer, Disabled Peoples' International, Asia Pacific Region, Bangkok

Franz Harsana Sasraningrad, executive council and regional leader for IDPA/DPI Indonesia, Yogyakarta, Indonesia

Leo C. W. Lam, chairperson, executive committee, Hong Kong Federation of Handicapped Youth, Kowloon, China

Charles Leung, chairperson, supervisory committee, Hong Kong Federation of Handicapped Youth; leader, Hong Kong Federation of the Blind, Hong Kong Island, China

Wiriya Namsiripongpun, past president Disabled Peoples' International (DPI)-Thailand; member, Association of the Blind of Thailand, Bangkok

Narong Patibatsarakich, director, Caulfield Memorial Library for the Blind; chairperson DPI-Thailand; Bangkok, Nonthaburi, Thailand

Jureeratana Pongpaew, librarian, board member DPI-Thailand, Bangkok

Pipat Prasatsuwan, executive council member, DPI-Thailand, Chiang Mai, Thailand

Koesbiono Sarmanhadi, associate secretary general, Persatuan Penyandang Cacat Indonesia (Indonesia Disabled Peoples' Association, IDPA), Jakarta, Indonesia

Dr. Rajinder Singh Sethi, coordinator, National Deaf-Blind League, Bombay, India

Padma Shri Dr. Rajendra T. Vyas, honorary general secretary, National Association for the Blind, Bombay, India

Europe

Rachel Hurst, chairperson, DPI-Europe; project director, Disability Awareness in Action, London, England

Adolph Ratzka, director, Institute on Independent Living, Stockholm, Sweden

PART I

Introduction

*When people with disabilities come to the conclusion that they
have the right to be in the community, to have a say in how that
community treats them, they are beginning to develop a
consciousness about taking control of their lives and resisting all
attempts to give others that control.*

Ed Roberts, founder and president,
World Institute on Disability

*We always emphasize the independent role of disabled
organizations and our movement. We do this because we must be
independent so we can criticize anyone, even the government.
The reason we stress the separate role of our organizations is that
we must advocate for ourselves, always. We should not rely on
political parties to liberate ourselves.*

Joshua Malinga, former chairperson,
Disabled Peoples' International,
general secretary, Southern Africa
Federation of the Disabled

CHAPTER 1

Nothing About Us Without Us

I first heard the expression "Nothing About Us Without Us" in South Africa in 1993. Michael Masutha and William Rowland, two leaders of Disabled People South Africa, separately invoked the slogan, which they had heard used by someone from Eastern Europe at an international disability rights conference. The slogan's power derives from its location of the source of many types of (disability) oppression and its simultaneous opposition to such oppression in the context of control and voice.

"Nothing About Us Without Us" resonates with the philosophy and history of the disability rights movement (DRM), a movement that has embarked on a belated mission parallel to other liberation movements. As Ed Roberts, one of the leading figures of the international DRM, has said, "If we have learned one thing from the civil rights movement in the U.S., it's that when others speak for you, you lose" (Driedger 1989:28). In this sense, "Our Bodies, Ourselves" and "Power to the People" can be recognized as precedents for "Nothing About Us Without Us." The DRM's demand for control is the essential theme that runs through all its work, regardless of political-economic or cultural differences. Control has universal appeal for DRM activists because the needs of people with disabilities and the potential for meeting these needs are everywhere conditioned by a dependency born of powerlessness, poverty, degradation, and institutionalization. This dependency, saturated with paternalism, begins with the onset of disability and continues until death. The condition of dependency is presently typical for hundreds of millions of people throughout the world.

Only in the past twenty-five years has this condition begun to change. Although little noticed and affecting only a small percentage of people with disabilities, this transformation is profound. For the first time in recorded human history politically active people with disabilities are beginning to proclaim that they know what is best for themselves and their community. This is a militant, revelational claim aptly capsulized in "Nothing About Us Without Us."

The Dialectics of Disability Oppression and Empowerment

Very little has been written on disability oppression and even less on the resistance to it. Furthermore, while there is a growing body of literature on disability in Europe and the United States, little information is available about disability in other parts of the world. What we know about disability—a significant part of the human condition—and hence about the human condition itself is thus fundamentally incomplete. I have undertaken such a discourse on disability. It is part descriptive, part conversational, part theoretical, and wholly argumentative. My thesis synthesizes theories and opinions about oppression and exploitation, power and ideology, resistance and empowerment. In the end, this book is as much a polemic, filtered by many voices and personal experiences, as anything else.

Chapters 2 through 6 explore the outrageous conditions in which hundreds of millions of people with disabilities live the world over—a reality that, unfortunately, cannot be contested. Beginning with chapter 7 I describe how some people with disabilities have organized to resist these conditions. Some might think any attempt to establish a comprehensive theory of disability oppression is preposterous, given the thousands of cultures and the political-economic disparities across the globe. These differences present many problems, but they are not, I believe, irreconcilable. One of the most important findings from interviews with more than fifty disability rights activists in ten countries is the similarity of lived disability experiences across cultures and political-economic zones. It is also clear that in the most disparate places the disability rights movement approaches and resists the particularities of the disability experience in very similar ways. Within this resistance lies the potential, however speculative and problematic, for the elimination of (disability) oppression. Simply put, this book is about the dialectics of the disability experience: oppression and its opposites, resistance and empowerment.

My mission is threefold. First, I wish to familiarize readers with an epistemological break with previous thinking about disability—a break that has affected millions of people with and without disabilities and that will even more widely influence people in the decades to come. Second, I intend to suggest ways of thinking about relationships and conditions of oppression and resistance that have rarely been applied to disability. In doing so, I attempt to answer, among other questions, why so many people acquiesce to oppression and why some people not only individually resist these conditions but also actively organize to change them. Third, I want to provide a political, economic, and cultural context to better *understand and support* an emerging international disability rights consciousness and movement. The point is not that every person with a disability experiences the same kind of oppression and identically resists it but rather that people with disabilities are oppressed and resist this oppression individually and collectively in ways that are generalizable.

My motivation is simple. I have seen and felt how people with disabilities are treated. In the most obvious and the subtlest ways, these conditions cry out for attention and are, in themselves, a fundamental critique of the existing world order. This book is not a plea for pity. We have had enough of that. It is also not an expression of hope for a helping hand. Hope is useful only when it is not illusory, and help is useful only when it leads to empowerment. *Nothing About Us Without Us* both advocates an epistemological break with old thinking about disability and demands an end to the cycles of dependency into which hundreds of millions of people with disabilities are forced.

Methodology and Other Considerations

This book is founded principally on the everyday life of people with disabilities. It derives first and foremost from my own particular experiences as a person with a disability and as an activist in the disability rights movement in the United States. Second, it comes out of others' experiences described in conversations, discussions, and interviews or excerpted from the existing literature. The "evidence" that follows is on one level self-reflection. We might call this method of observation "human sensuous practice" or "lessons from life." I would argue that these experiences so closely coincide that they can be synthesized into a general, albeit partial, description of everyday life for people with disabilities.

Most of these lessons from life come from the Third World. To consider disability oppression as a generalized phenomenon, attention must be directed to those parts of the world where 80 percent of all people (with disabilities) live. To do this, I have used the analysis and personal stories of disability rights activists from these regions, along with those of activists and political theorists from other parts of the world. The political-economic and sociocultural dimensions of disability oppression, as well as peoples' resistance and organization, are framed by these narratives.

Concerns and Limitations

It should be emphasized from the outset that this book rests on what Eric Hobsbawm called "curiously uneven foundations" in the preface to his book *The Age of Extremes*. Although I believe the everyday lives of people with different disabilities in different cultures have many common qualities and characteristics, I also know there are serious limitations my general exposition has to acknowledge. Many important geopolitical and cultural areas of the world are not covered in this study, among them, most prominently, northern Asia (Japan, Korea, the People's Republic of China [PRC]) and the Middle East. My understanding of Europe, especially eastern and southern Europe, is also limited. Some aspects of Chinese culture are picked up in interviews with the Chinese DRM leaders in Hong Kong (and in secondary sources), but the reach of the PRC's political, economic, and social influences is not shown. Cultures of the Middle East are not accounted for, although Moslem views and attitudes toward disability are partially covered in examining Indonesia and consulting secondary sources. I cannot say if Indonesian practices resemble those of the Arab Middle East.

In addition, many types of disabilities are not sufficiently represented. The absence of people with mental and cognitive disabilities is especially notable because these disabilities combine to make up the largest disability "category." Although I have incorporated some material from U.S. sources, it is sketchy. Still, I received almost universal confirmation from disability rights activists that people with mental illness are the most discriminated against and the most isolated in their respective countries. This is a significant finding.

Also meriting fuller representation are people who are deaf. Their isolation, especially in the Third World, parallels that of individuals with mental disabilities. The scarcity of sign language interpreters exacerbates this condition and also compounds the difficulty of identifying and interviewing even those who are politically active.

Finally, I have set the topic of AIDS aside to narrow the scope of this project. To be sure, in many countries and regions—indeed throughout Africa, Brazil, and possibly Thailand as well—one can reasonably argue that AIDS is the most important disability issue. There is no doubt that the ideological and social experiences of people with AIDS closely parallel those of people with other disabilities, especially disabilities closely linked with "illness"—cancer, mental illness, diabetes, and so on. Susan Sontag's two brilliant expositions on the "feelings" embodied in and the imagery associated with various disabilities, *Illness as Metaphor* and *AIDS and Its Metaphors,* are applicable. General economic and specific sociocultural similarities do, however, unify the experience of disability. We realize this almost intuitively. Besides the ubiquitous conditions of poverty and degradation that surround it, we know that when a person becomes disabled, she or he immediately becomes "less"—what Wilhelm Reich refers to as "bio-energetic shrinking." This is the phenomenon Sontag explores in *Illness as Metaphor* and is the thought most associated with disability per se. A person goes to a physician to get a routine physical exam. After the procedure, the physician, noticeably different in demeanor, announces that the "patient" has cancer. The person immediately feels sick (sometimes referred to as a sinking feeling) and shrinks. *They become less,* although there is nothing different from moments before, when the person felt healthy and full. The psychosocial manifestation of this phenomenon unifies all disabilities, from cancer and AIDS to spinal cord injury and amputation to deafness and blindness.

Terminology, Definitions, and Statistics

Now we come to questions of terminology and definition. The first term requiring definition is "disability." For my purposes, disability is based on social and functional criteria. This means, first, that disability is not a medical category but a social one. Disability is socially constructed. For example, if a particular culture treats a person as having a disability, the person has one. Second, the category "disability" includes people with socially defined functional limitations. For instance, deaf people are considered disabled although many deaf individuals insist they do not have a disability. People do not get to choose whether they have disabilities. Most political activists would define disability as a condition imposed on individuals by society. This definition is mirrored in the Americans with Disabilities Act of 1990: "The term 'disability' means with respect to an individual (a) a physical or mental impairment that substantially limits one or more of the major life activities of such individual; (b) a record of such an impairment; (c) being regarded as having such an impairment."

Estimates of the numbers of disabled persons based on this definition (broadly considered) have been available for twenty years and have not changed much. Writing in *Rehabilitation International* in 1981, John H. Noble, Jr., stated, "In 1975 people throughout the world suffering [*sic*] all types and degrees of disability numbered an estimated 490 million (12.3 percent of the world population); by the year 2000, their number will reach an estimated 846 million (13 percent). Whereas in 1975 more than three-quarters of this population lived in developing countries, by the year 2000 more than four-fifths of all disabled people will live in these countries." Ten years later, the U.S. General Accounting Office quoted the United Nations as estimating that 80 percent of the world's 500 million persons with disabilities live in the "developing countries" (the UN's term). In the 1995 UNESCO report, "Overcoming Obstacles to the Integration of Disabled People," England's Disability Awareness in Action breaks this number out further: 300 million people with disabilities live in Asia (70 million children); 50 million in Africa; and 34 million in Latin America.

The second term needing clarification is "oppression." Oppression occurs when individuals are *systematically* subjected to political, economic, cultural, or social degradation because they belong to a social group. Oppression of people results from structures of domination and subordination and, correspondingly, ideologies of superiority and inferiority. In *Justice and the Politics of Difference,* Iris Young presents five "faces" of oppression: exploitation, oppression that takes place in the process of labor; marginalization, the inability or unwillingness of the economic system to incorporate a group of people in its political, economic, and cultural life; powerlessness, a group's lack of power or authority; cultural imperialism, the demeaning of a group by the dominant culture's values; and violence, random or organized attacks on a group (1990:48–65). These categories, if interpreted correctly, are helpful in defining oppression.

Most important, oppression, like all social processes, must be understood as experienced in and conditioned by real life. Political, economic, and cultural contexts determine the similarities and differences in the experience of people with disabilities.

Two other terms that require definition or at least an explanation are "underdeveloped countries" and "Third World." These terms are intertwined, and many people do not much like them. Analogous terms or phrases include "transitional societies," "developing countries," "undeveloped countries," "the periphery," and "newly industrialized countries." All of these mean different things to different people. I prefer "underdeveloped" because it implies the process colonies went through as colonizers expropriated and exploited the cheap labor and resources available there. These countries and regions were *under*developed. In my use, "underdevelopment" denotes the expropriation and despoliation of huge chunks of what has come to be known as the Third World. Some prefer the term "maldevelopment." Both locate the root causes of the political-economic circumstances of these regions in colonialism and imperialism without casting aspersions on the region's people, although both recognize the collusion of indigenous elites. This is my intent as well. Many prefer to use the term "developing countries." The problem, of course, is that most, if not all, are not developing. They are, and have long been, stagnating in crisis. It is important to remember that "underdevelopment" is a political-economic condition and does not imply anything about history and culture. Economically poor countries have exceptionally rich cultures and histories.

And finally, I use the terms "Third World" and "periphery" to position Latin America, Africa, and Asia and parts of the Middle East in relation to the first (the United States) and second worlds (Japan and Europe) in the context of political economy. In the past, some people divided the first and second worlds between the capitalist and socialist worlds, but that division is now unnecessary. Significant political-economic divisions do, however, separate the United States from the rest of the world because of its military superiority. Some people have suggested the term "Fourth World" for those nations whose national economies generate less than $1,000 per capita. This is splitting hairs. All nations of the Third World are poor whether they are at the low or high end of the economic range (most often cited as $200 to $4,000 per capita). I use the terms "Third World" and "periphery" interchangeably because both imply an economic center and an economic periphery.

On Theory

Finally, a comment on theoretical work itself. However well formulated, I believe that any theory of oppression and responses to it can only provide a partial explanation. There are, of course, theoretical breakthroughs. And it is my hope to contribute a few bricks to the construction of a comprehensive theory. It cannot be otherwise. Disability oppression, like all kinds of oppression, is complex and multileveled. Disability oppression is itself most often a partial experience of oppression. People with disabilities experience other crucial kinds of oppression based on class, race, and gender. These are undoubtedly profound influences on the particularities of the lived experiences of people with disabilities, regardless of place. A literature has begun in some of these areas, as I try to note in passing. Acknowledging these severe limitations, I have pressed on. For it seems to me that while we can debate the extent, if any, to which rich white men with disabilities are oppressed, the more critical questions involve how the hundreds of millions of poor people with disabilities are surviving and what it will take for them to have lives of dignity and independence.

The Lived Experiences of Disability and the Transformation of Consciousness

As noted earlier, a remarkable and unprecedented paradigm shift has recently occurred which represents a historic break with the traditional perception of disability as a sick, abnormal, and pathetic condition. This shift poses a fundamental challenge to the ideological oppression of people with disabilities. For it sees disability as normal, not inferior, and demands self-determination over the resources people with disabilities need. This new perspective unfolds out of a changing world in which a relatively few political activists with disabilities are challenging the old ways of thinking about and treating disability. The stories of these people provide compelling evidence for the basis and direction of this paradigm shift. Because the lived experiences of people with disabilities are critical to my success in explaining this paradigm shift and in developing a broad thesis of oppression and resistance, I will present throughout this book short excerpts from the extensive interviews I conducted over the course of a decade. The excerpts below condense crucial influences in the life of two activists, Joshua Malinga, former chairperson of Disabled Peoples' International and the general secretary of the Southern Africa Federation of the Disabled, and Rosangela Berman Bieler, president of South America's first center for independent living in Rio de Janeiro and a leading activist in Brazil's disability rights movement since 1980. They are included here to indicate the nature of the interviews themselves and to begin the juxtaposition of lived oppression versus the transformation of consciousness into active resistance.

Jim Charlton (J.C.): "I am interested in the relation between disability oppression and the political consciousness of disability rights activists. Specifically, I am interested in your personal history and why it is that you have become a political activist."

Joshua Malinga: "I was born in 1944 about 100 kilometers from Bulawayo. As you know, we in Zimbabwe have two homes, in our village and also in the city where we must go to find work. My father was a village chief and had six wives and thirty-eight children. I was the only one to get polio. . . . From early on, all my brothers and sisters went off to school and I had to stay home to scare away the animals from our house and do errands. . . . Everything I am now, it's all because of accidents of fortune. In 1956, the first accident of fortune occurred. One of my brothers broke his arm and found himself in the hospital. There, my brother met this man, Jauros Jiri, who was developing a social service network which now is a very big charity agency of twenty-five to thirty institutions. After this discussion, my brother told Jauros Jiri about me, so Jauros Jiri organized for me to come to the institution. Although my parents didn't want me to go, there was obviously nothing at home for me. I was very young (13) but had never been to school, so all this was very new. Jauros Jiri began to train me in leathercraft and I had some classes for reading and math. Their only idea for me was to be a cobbler. In 1959, there was another accident of fortune for me. In that year, Jauros Jiri received money from the government to bring in a trained teacher. This teacher noticed that education was easy for me, and he encouraged me to go to school. Although the people at the institution didn't want me to go because this teacher within the institution was the one encouraging me, it was hard for them to stop me. . . . Even from day one,

I had an inborn attitude not to accept the attitudes at the institution. These ideas were very bad. For example, disabled people were told when to eat, when to sleep, that they couldn't make love, it was banned. . . . Especially in the period 1965–1967, I had a growing consciousness about disability.

By the mid-1970s I and a few others wanted to reject all these ideas and start our own organization. By 1965, I began organizing disabled people because I knew things were not right. First, we called ourselves Inmates Representative Council and then Trainees Representatives Council. Later, we became Council for the Welfare of the Disabled and then National Council for the Welfare of the Disabled. . . . In fact, I was the first Jauros Jiri person to go through primary and secondary school. Then I went to technical college and was probably the first black to go to technical college in Bulawayo. . . . When I left college I could not get a job except at the Jauros Jiri institution. My jobs escalated there from accountant to bookkeeper to administrator of the biggest Jauros Jiri project. When I left in 1980, I was the CEO of Jauros Jiri. . . . At that time, another accident of fortune occurred.

The year 1980 was an important one because at this time Zimbabwe became independent. At this time a fellow from the international development foundation OXFAM visited the Jauros Jiri institution to see about funding their programs. In the meeting, I could tell he didn't want to fund a charity. I think he was mostly interested in development, not services. So anyway, during the meeting I slipped him a note asking could he meet me after the meeting and he said okay. So when I met him, I told him that I detected he had some reservations about the Jauros Jiri institution, and I told him about a disability group I was involved with, that we were starting to organize but had no funds. That we had to take paper and other materials where we could and that we needed an office and secretary and some other things. I told him OXFAM should fund us because we were interested in civil rights and changing the world. He said okay again. Then I said that I knew about this upcoming international conference in Canada and could he find funds for me to go. This did happen, and I went to Winnipeg to attend the Rehabilitation International [RI] Conference. . . .

As you know, 1981 was the International Year of Disabled Persons, a year dedicated to full participation of disabled persons. But RI didn't really practice this. At the conference, there were 5,000 delegates but only 200 disabled persons. So the disabled delegates got together and demanded that the executive committee be 50 percent people with disabilities. This was overwhelmingly rejected, so there was a split and the 200 disabled persons and some others formed Disabled Peoples' International, of which I have held various posts. I am the current chairperson until 1994. When I returned I was a changed person. When I left I was very passive, but when I returned I was very radical. Immediately when I returned from Winnipeg in 1981 we changed our name from National Council for the Welfare of the Disabled to the National Council of Disabled Persons Zimbabwe. At that time, we began to recognize that disability was about human rights, about social change, about organizing ourselves. We did not want to emphasize welfare but organization."

Rosangela Berman Bieler: "I was in a car accident in 1976 when I was 19 years old. I was at the university studying journalism. As a quadriplegic, I was involved in rehabilitation for over a year. I became aware of disability rights because I had very good peer counselors who helped me avoid feeling pity for myself and to feel part of a group. We went to bars and movies together. In those years, it was very unusual to see someone using a wheelchair in the streets of Rio, but five or six people together using wheelchairs was shocking, it was a revolution. The peer counseling was very, very important to me. . . . Before my accident, I was a very active teenager. I played the guitar, went to bars, came home early in the morning, had lots of friends. My accident was a big change for me initially until I met those friends I was talking about. The university was very inaccessible so my family helped build ramps into the buildings. . . . I had my own consciousness about disability, but it was also part of the larger political movement of the country. . . . I started organizing at the rehabilitation center because I wanted to travel, do sports, and other social things. In 1979, we had our first meeting to discuss building a national organization and talk about what we would do for 1980. In those years, we had slightly more freedom to organize so we had to take advantage of it. There were many things going on at this time, especially among students. For example, I was involved in political activities as a representative of an art school in the student movement in 1982. All of my political consciousness was through the student movement. Each member of the student movement had to develop his or her own area. Mine was disability. In 1982 we had our first elections in the country. I was active in the Workers Party [PT] as a representative of students and painters. We were very organized and militant."

J.C.: "How do attitudes and myths about disability get expressed in your country? I'm interested in how the political and cultural aspects of everyday life are connected. What are the prevailing attitudes today toward disability? Have you seen changes in attitudes over time? And are there differences between rural and urban areas?"

Joshua Malinga: "Now in Africa we have very backward ideas about disability. This is especially connected to witchcraft in the rural areas and to life as an oppressed people historically. . . . To be disabled in Zimbabwe, people think you are not a full human being. Our activities are not considered normal, you aren't expected to play an adult role. We have a long way to go, although small changes can be seen. We began to target attitudes in 1981 because attitudes were key. To this end, we knew that we had to mobilize and organize people with disabilities. . . . Negative attitudes brought about charities, not movements, and when you talk about changing attitudes you don't limit yourself to legislation; it can be an instrument but only that."

Rosangela Berman Bieler: "The main characteristics of Brazilian culture are that it is paternalistic and it has a history of Portuguese colonialism. Brazil has incredible contrasts which have to be taken into account when analyzing the question of how paternalism works. For example, the south of Brazil was colonized by the Germans. It's like another country. Paternalism influences the way people think about disability. The church has an important role in promoting it as well as the military dictatorship. Much of our situation in Brazil, the social problems, the poverty, and the apathy, is because of the military dictatorship. The dictatorship had a powerful role in the ideas of my generation and that of my father. This shows up in the lack of political leadership in Brazil. Very few people wanted to become involved in politics for about fifteen years. People were scared, and this limited the number of people with political experience. Also, many of the really good political leaders were killed or went into exile. . . . However, the problems of paternalism existed before the dictatorship. In spite of European colonization, we have more identification with the Americans than with the Europeans. So our backward attitudes are much more tied to the Latin American stereotypes. Paternalism has also affected us in the sense that disabled people do not have a habit of self-organization. . . . I would say that Rio is very liberated and open-minded. This made it easier for me as a teenager and as a young adult dealing with my disability. Everyone talks about sex and sexuality. I think it is easier for us who have disabilities in Brazil to be able to discuss and figure these kinds of things out. In fact, I think more women with disabilities are marrying in Brazil than in other countries I have visited."

J.C.: "What kinds of organizations are there of people with disabilities, what kinds of political philosophies and tactics do they have, and what has been your personal experience with them?"

Rosangela Berman Bieler: "We began organizing at the rehab center. We put out newsletters such as *Camino* [trend, path] and *Clandestino* [clandestine]. The latter was a play on words because we called our disability group The Clan. The political meetings in those years were fantastic for me because I was involved from the beginning. I was in leadership at national and international levels. We also worked on a newsletter, *Etapa,* for our national organization. This was an information newsletter mostly. We had 12,000 people on our subscription list. We got money from advertisers. Everybody worked for free. . . . During this time, many people with disabilities who were active had a real catharsis. We developed a politics and a form of organization that had never existed in Brazil before. By 1983, there was a strong national organization. In the beginning, I was very radical. That has changed somewhat. I was radical in the sense that I did not want to cooperate with any institution that dealt with disability. I also believed only people with disabilities should vote at assemblies and meetings. Now I believe leadership should be disabled, but there is a role for the able-bodied.

We need a broader unity. . . . Now I represent Rehabilitation International for Latin America. Its history was to speak for the disabled. Really RI speaks for professionals, but they must adapt to the new conditions they are trying to influence. They have even elected a paraplegic as president who also represents New Zealand. An irony for me in this regard is that the person who preceded me as vice president for Latin America in RI was the same doctor who kicked me and my friends out of the rehabilitation center for organizing. . . . I have changed my attitudes about the movement in many regards recently. That is why I started the CIL [center for independent living] in Rio. I gave twelve years of my life to the national movement. Personal competition among disability leaders was very discouraging. I know this happened in many countries. I just became disgusted with the in-fighting. *Etapa* was very important for many people. For the first time, that newsletter brought information about disability to the rural areas. We worked on *Etapa* for eight years. . . . I feel fortunate that through my disability work I was able to visit many countries and get to know many disability rights activists. I went to Maryland where I visited CILs. I had never heard of independent living before my trip to Maryland. When other people decided to stop working on *Etapa*, I could no longer work in that movement so I, along with a few other people, formed the Rio CIL."

J.C.: "Can you talk about what's going on in the region? Where is disability rights strongest?"

Joshua Malinga: "When I came back from Winnipeg I was assigned to organize the region of Africa. We Zimbabweans have impacted the organizations of disabled people throughout southern Africa. I believe in South Africa they have as strong a movement as we have in Zimbabwe. Probably because of the struggle against apartheid the disabled community is more politicized, so it has progressed well. The newest is in Angola. It was the hardest to organize because of the destabilization there by South Africa and the American government. Of course, 90 percent of our problems in the region are directly related to the role of the United States. In Mozambique, an organization was formed three years ago which is very organized, although it was difficult as well, similar to Angola. I think the ruling party played a role. We always emphasize the independent role of disabled organizations and our movement from the government. This is the problem we are presently experiencing in Namibia, as in Mozambique, where most of the disabled people we are working with are ex-combatants who are very close to or in the ruling party. So our task is to break that relationship up. We do this because we must be independent so we can criticize anyone, even the government. The reason we stress the separate role of our organizations is that we must advocate for ourselves, always. We should not rely on political parties to liberate ourselves. Our progress in all the countries is uneven. . . . We have many barriers, but the most important is the level of development in the region. But we have no proof about social systems. All governments treat disabled people badly. They all see us as a burden. All governments, whether socialist or capitalist, have separated us from the rest of society. By the end of the day, people are judged by their own activity. Until we are businessmen, politicians, community leaders, people at all levels of society, we will be marginalized and segregated."

The sea change we are witnessing in the disabled community is embodied in and epitomized by disability rights activists like Joshua Malinga and Rosangela Berman Bieler. Whereas people with disabilities have always struggled to survive, many are now struggling to change their world as well. The replacement of the false consciousness of self-pity and helplessness with the raised consciousness of dignity, anger, and empowerment has meaningfully affected the way in which many people with disabilities relate personally and politically to society. The personal histories of each of the people I interviewed, in different ways and for different reasons, show raised consciousness as the real appreciation of one's self, one's own image, values, and interests, and not the manufactured images and projected values and interests of the dominant culture. In later chapters, I further track the development from raised consciousness to empowered consciousness, a kind of consciousness that involves a commitment on the part of the individual to act on his or her raised consciousness. There are many people with disabilities who have raised consciousness, but there are few who are politically active, who are committed to empowering others. These people are organizers, agitators, and educators who make up the disability rights movement.

Nothing About Us Without Us: The Politics and Organization of Empowerment

The disability rights movement is not unlike other new and important social movements demanding self-representation and control over the resources needed to live a decent life. Two years after hearing the slogan "Nothing About Us Without Us" in South Africa, I noticed on the front page of the Mexico City daily *La Jornada* a picture of thousands of landless peasants marching under the banner "Nunca Mas Sin Nosotros" (Never Again Without Us) (March 19, 1995). At that moment I began using *Nothing About Us Without Us* as my working title.

People with disabilities have formed a wide array of organizations to respond to political and personal needs. Each organization has its own motivation and agenda, lines of communication and leadership, and expectations and scope. These range from small political action and self-help groups, social clubs, and income-generating initiatives to large national and regional federations or coalitions of disability-related groups. These organizations, given their specific circumstances and histories, have developed strategies and patterns of organization that in a very short time have advanced the overall progress of their communities. They have promoted an increased identification with others who have disabilities and an interest in what many have come to call "disability culture." The slogan "Nothing About Us Without Us" captures the essence of these developments for a number of reasons. First, to understand anything about people with disabilities or the disability rights movement, one must recognize their individual and collective necessities. "Nothing About Us Without Us" forces people to think about the broad implications of "nothing" in various political-economic and cultural contexts. Second, a growing number of people with disabilities have developed a consciousness that transforms the notion and concept of disability from a medical condition to a political and social condition. "Nothing About Us Without Us" requires people with disabilities to recognize their need to control and take responsibility for their own lives. It also forces political-economic and cultural systems to incorporate people with disabilities into the decision-making process and to recognize that the experiential knowledge of these people is pivotal in making decisions that affect their lives. Third, while the number of people affected by this epistemological breakthrough is relatively small, a movement has emerged. The disability rights movement has developed its own ideology and politics. It is a liberation movement that is confronting the realpolitik of the world at large. The demand "Nothing About Us Without Us" is a demand for self-determination and a necessary precedent to liberation. Fourth, the philosophy and organization that the international DRM embraces includes independence and integration, empowerment and human rights, and self-help and self-determination. The demand "Nothing About Us Without Us" affirms the essence of these principles. Finally, the DRM is one of many emerging movements in which new attitudes and worldviews are being created. Through its struggle comes a vision that requires a fundamental reordering of priorities and resources. "Nothing About Us Without Us" suggests such a sea change in the way disability oppression is conceived and resisted.

PART II

Disability Oppression and Everyday Life

When discussing disability, we must take into consideration the grave social and economic problems afflicting Brazil's people. The country suffers from misery and malnutrition, as well as the lack of prevention, education, and sanitation, among other problems. In this country, where social injustice is represented by unfair distribution of income, 1 percent of the population is richer than all of the poor and 60 percent of the inhabitants earn only US $40 a week. This is why the majority of the 15 million people with disabilities in Brazil are in pitiful condition. Lacking resources and information, with survival as their main battle, they are forgotten by their families, the community and competent authorities. They are outcasts *deprived of social life, dignity, and citizenship.*

Rosangela Berman Bieler, president, Center
for Independent Living, Rio de Janeiro

CHAPTER 2

The Dimensions of
Disability Oppression

An Overview

The vast majority of people with disabilities have always been poor, powerless, and degraded. Disability oppression is a product of both the past and the present. Some aspects of disability oppression are remnants of ancien régimes of politics and economics, customs and beliefs, and others can be traced to more recent developments. To understand the consequences and implications for people with disabilities an analysis is called for which considers how the overarching structures of society influence this trend. This is especially relevant in light of the United Nations' contention that their condition is worsening: "Handicapped people remain *outcasts* around the world, living in shame and squalor among populations lacking not only in resources to help them but also in understanding. And with their numbers growing rapidly, their plight is getting worse. . . . The normal perception is that nothing can be done for disabled children. This has to do with prejudice and old-fashioned thinking that this punishment comes from God, some evil spirits or magic. . . . We have a catastrophic human rights situation. . . . They [disabled persons] are a group without power."[1]

There is a great deal to say about disability oppression, not only because it is complex and multifaceted but also because we have so little experience conceptualizing its phenomenology and logic. Until very recently most analyses of why people with disabilities have been and continue to be poor, powerless, and degraded have been mired in an anachronistic academic tradition that understands the "status" of people with disabilities in terms of deviance and stigma. This has been compounded by the lack of participation by people with disabilities in these analyses. Fortunately, this has begun to change. Disability rights activists have recently undertaken important and fruitful efforts to frame disability oppression. These projects, however insightful, have been limited by their scope and inability to account for the systemic nature of disability oppression. For example, in the article "Malcolm Teaches Us, Too," in the *Disability Rag*, Marta Russell writes,

Malcolm's most important message was to love blackness, to love black culture. Malcolm insisted that loving blackness itself was an act of resistance in a white dominated society. By exposing the internalized racial self-hatred that deeply penetrated the psyches of U.S. colonized black people, Malcolm taught that blacks could decolonize their minds by coming to blackness to be spiritually renewed, transformed. He believed that, only then, could blacks unite to gain the equality they rightfully deserved. . . . It is equally important for disabled persons to recognize what it means to live as a disabled person in a physicalist society—that is, one which places its value on physical agility. When our bodies do not work like able-bodied person's bodies, we're disvalued. Our oppression by able-bodied persons is rife with the message: There is something wrong, something "defective" with us—because we have a disability. . . . We must identify with ourselves and others like us. Like Malcolm sought for his race, disabled persons must build a culture which will unify us and enable us to gain our human rights. (1994:11–12)

There is much of value for the DRM in what Russell says. She is patently correct, for instance, to point people with disabilities toward Malcolm X in terms of recognition and identity, self-hatred and self-respect. But she, like Malcolm X, is wrong on the question of where the basis of oppression lies. Both identify oppression with the Other, a view that is quite prevalent among disability rights activists. For Russell, the Other is able-bodied people; for Malcolm, it was white people (although he began to change this view shortly before his assassination). Both situate oppression in the realm of the ideas of others and not in systems or structures that marginalize people for political-economic and sociocultural reasons. As the great Mexican novelist Julio Cortazar writes in *Hopscotch*, "Nothing can be denounced if the denouncing is done within the system that belongs to the thing denounced" ([1966]1987: chap. 99). My project then is as much a polemic directed at the disability rights movement as at a more general public. My point to other activists is that the logic of disability oppression closely parallels the oppression of other groups. It is a logic bound up with political-economic needs and belief systems of domination. From these priorities and values has evolved a world system dominated by the laws of capital and profit and the ethos of individualism and image worship. This point is just as important as my call to the general public, especially the international community, to recognize and respond to an extraordinary human rights tragedy, what former UN Secretary General Javier Perez de Cuellar once called "the silent emergency."

Political Economy and the World System

Political economy is crucial in constructing a theory of disability oppression because poverty and powerlessness are cornerstones of the dependency people with disabilities experience. As the social science of how politics and economics influence and limit everyday life, political economy is primarily concerned with issues of class because class positions groups of people in relation to economic production and exchange, political power and privilege. Today, class not only structures the political and economic relationships between the worker, peasant, farmer, intellectual, small-scale entrepreneur, government bureaucrat, army general, banker, and industrialist, it mediates family and community life insofar as relationships exist in these which affect people's economic viability.[2] In political-economic terms, everyday life is informed by where and how individuals, families, and communities are incorporated into a world system dominated by the few who control the means of production and force. This has been the case for a long time. The logic of this system regulates and explains who survives and prospers, who controls and who is controlled, and, not simply metaphorically, who is on the inside and who is on the outside (of power).

Perhaps the most fitting characterization of the socioeconomic condition of people with disabilities is that they are outcasts. This is how they are portrayed in the UN report cited at the beginning of this chapter. It was also repeated by many of the disability rights activists I interviewed. It seems reasonable to ask, why is this depiction so common? The answer is two-sided, sociocultural and political-economic. On one side are the panoply of reactionary and iconoclastic attitudes about disability. These are addressed briefly in the next section and in depth in chapter 4. On the other side stands a political-economic formation that does not need and in fact cannot accommodate a vast group of people in its production, exchange, and reproduction. Put differently, people with disabilities, like many others, are preponderantly part of a worldwide phenomenon that James O'Connor called "surplus population" (1973:161)[3] and Istvan Meszaros called "superfluous people" (1995:702).

The extent and implications of this phenomenon are experienced differently. For example, it is readily apparent that people, even those with disabilities, living in the more economically developed regions of the world have higher "standards of living" than their counterparts in the Third World. The United States and Europe have safety nets that catch "outcasts" before their very livelihoods are called into question. This is not necessarily the case in the Third World.

The 300 million to 400 million people with disabilities who live in the periphery, like the vast majority of people in those regions, exist in abject poverty, but I would go further and argue that, for social and cultural reasons, their lives are even more difficult. These are the poorest and most powerless people on earth.

As the global economy developed, it created more than just the wandering gypsies of southern Europe and the *posseiros* (squatters) of South America. It created an enormous number of outcasts who must be set apart from what Karl Marx called the "reserve army of labor"—a resource to be tapped in times of economic expansion (although Marx uses them interchangeably in *Grundrisse* [1973:491]). For hundreds of millions of outcasts—beggars and others who depend on charity for survival; prostitutes, drug dealers, and others who survive through criminal activities; the homeless, refugees, and others forced to live somewhere besides their home or homeland;[4] and many others—will seldom, if ever, under ordinary circumstances be used in the production, exchange, and distribution of political and economic goods and services. They are essentially declassed. So many people fall into this category that U.S. economists have created the category "underclass" to refer to them. The UN has even created the preposterous category "admissible levels of poverty" to describe the condition of the best-off among these people.

People with disabilities, at least as a group, may have been the first to join the ranks of the underclass. Since feudalism and even earlier, they have lived outside the economy and political process.[5] It should be noted, of course, that few people with physical disabilities survived for very long in precapitalist economies.

The emergence and development of capitalism had an extraordinarily profound and positive impact on people with disabilities. For the first time, probably in the mid-1700s in parts of Europe, people living outside the spheres of production and exchange, the "surplus people," could rely on others to survive. Family members and friends who could accumulate more than the barest minimum necessary for survival had the "luxury" of being able to care for others. A century later the political-economic conditions were such that charities, which supported a large number of people, were established. Those who were cared for by these charities most often were the mentally ill, the blind, the alcoholic, the chronically ill. My analysis throughout this book centers on the political-economic and sociocultural relationships born out of these times and how they have developed differently in different economic zones and in different cultures. Essentially, I will argue, as Audre Lorde does in *Sister Outsider,* that these formations now not only stand as barriers to progress but also are the basis for peoples' oppression: "Institutionalized rejection of *difference* is an absolute necessity in a profit economy which needs outsiders as surplus people. As members of such an economy, we have *all* been programmed to respond to the human differences between us with fear and loathing and to handle that difference in one of three ways: ignore it, and if that is not possible, copy it if we think it is dominant, or destroy it if we think it is subordinate. But we have no patterns for relating across our human differences as equals. As a result, those differences have been misnamed and misused in the service of separation and confusion" (1984:77).

Culture(s) and Belief Systems

The modern world is composed of thousands of cultures, each with its own ways of thinking about other people, nature, family and community, social phenomena, and so on. Culture is sustained through customs, rituals, mythology, signs and symbols, and institutions such as religion and the mass media. Each of these informs the beliefs and attitudes that contribute to disability oppression. These attitudes are almost universally pejorative. They hold that people with disabilities are pitiful and that disability itself is abnormal. This is one of the social norms used to separate people with disabilities through classification systems that encompass education, housing, transportation, health care, and family life.

For early anthropologists, "culture" meant how values were attached to belief systems (Kroeber and Kluckhorn 1952:180–182). Since then the meaning of the term "culture" has become so contested that some have argued for its abandonment. Others consider it simply a "lived experience" or "lived antagonistic experiences." For Clifford Geertz, one of anthropology's preeminent theorists, the "culture concept . . . denotes a historically transmitted pattern of meanings embodied in symbols, a system of inherited conceptions expressed in symbolic forms by means of which men communicate, perpetuate, and develop their knowledge and attitudes toward life" (1973:89). Geertz's theory has many adherents, but it has also garnered its share of criticism, most commonly that it neglects the influence of politics and power. In *Ideology and Modern Culture*, John Thompson postulates a more reasonable position. Thompson's formulation is that the study of symbols as a way to interpret cultures must be done contextually, by recognizing that power relations order the experiences of everyday life in which these signs and symbols are produced, transmitted, and received:

The symbolic conception is a suitable starting point for the development of a constructive approach to the study of cultural phenomena. But the weakness of this conception—in the form it appears, for instance, in the writings of Geertz—is that it gives insufficient attention to the structured social relations within which symbols and symbolic actions are always embedded. Hence, I formulate what I call the structural conception of culture. Cultural phenomena, according to this conception, may be understood as symbolic forms in structured contexts, and cultural analysis may be construed as the study of the meaningful constitution and social contextualization of symbolic forms. (1990:123)

My notion of culture(s) is similar to Thompson's. Contrary to many traditions in anthropology, cultures are not independent or static formations. They interface and interact in the everyday world with history, politics and power, economic conditions and institutions, and nature. To neglect these important influences seems to miss important interstices where culture happens, is expressed, and, most important, is experienced. The point is not that one culture makes people do or think this and another that but that ideas and beliefs are informed by and in cultures and that cultures are partial expressions of a world in which the dualities of domination/subordination, superiority/inferiority, normality/abnormality are relentlessly reinforced and legitimized. Anthropologists may be able to find obscure cultures in which these dualities are not determinant, but this does not minimize their overarching influence.

The essential problem of recent anthropological work on culture and disability is that it perpetuates outmoded beliefs and continues to distance research from lived oppression. Contributors to Benedicte Ingstad and Susan Reynolds Whyte's *Disability and Culture* seem to be oblivious to the extraordinary poverty and degradation of people with disabilities. The book does add to our understanding of how the conceptualization and symbolization of disability takes place, but its language and perspective are still lodged in the past. In the first forty pages alone we find the words *suffering, lameness, interest group, incapacitated, handicapped, deformities.* Notions of oppression, dominant culture, justice, human rights, political movement, and self-determination are conspicuously absent. We can read hundreds of pages without even contemplating degradation. Unlike these anthropologists and of course many others, my thesis is that backward attitudes about disability are not the basis for disability oppression, disability oppression is the basis for backward attitudes.

(False) Consciousness and Alienation

The third component of disability oppression is its psychological internalization. This creates a (false) consciousness and alienation that divides people and isolates individuals. Most people with disabilities actually come to believe they are less normal, less capable than others. Self-pity, self-hate, shame, and other manifestations of this process are devastating for they prevent people with disabilities from knowing their real selves, their real needs, and their real capabilities and from recognizing the options they in fact have. False consciousness and alienation also obscure the source of their oppression. They cannot recognize that their self-perceived pitiful lives are simply a perverse mirroring of a pitiful world order. In this regard people with disabilities have much in common with others who also have internalized their own oppression. Marx called this "the self-annihilation of the worker" and Frantz Fanon "the psychic alienation of the colonized." In *Femininity and Domination,* Sandra Lee Bartky exposes the roles of alienation, narcissism, and shame in the oppression of women. Each of these examples highlights the centrality of consciousness to any discussion of oppression. Consciousness, like culture, means different things to different people. Carl Jung said it is "everything that is not unconscious." Sartre said "consciousness is being" or "being-in-itself." For the Egyptian novelist Naguib Moufouz, it is "an awareness of the concealed side." Recently there have been attempts to develop a neurobiological theory of consciousness, the best known of which is Gerald Edelman's *The Remembered Present* (1989).

Whole philosophical systems and schools of psychology are built on the concept of consciousness. Appropriately, most postulate stages or types, even archetypes of consciousness. For Jung, everything important was interior, was "thought." The highest consciousness was individuation, or self-realization (the "summit"). This required gaining command of all four thought functions: sensation, feeling, thinking, and intuition. When one arrives at the intersection of these functions, "one opens one's eyes" (Campbell 1988:xxvi–xxx).

Marxism typically understood consciousness as metaphorical spirals of practice (experience) and theory (thought) intertwined. These spirals move incrementally, quantitatively. Consciousness, however, is not a linear progression. At points this quantitative buildup congeals into a "rupture," or a qualitative or transformational leap to another stage of consciousness where another spiral-like phenomenon begins. Consciousness can leap from being-in-itself (existence as is) to being-for-itself (consciously desiring change), Marx's equivalent of a leap in self-realization. While Jung's and, before him, Freud's great contribution to modern psychology was the discovery of the importance of the unconscious, their systems excluded political and social conditions. They were asocial and apolitical. This is where idealism (e.g., Jung, Hegel) and materialism (e.g., Marx, Sartre) split most dramatically. Sartre's withering critique of psychology began with this difference. According to Sartre, "the Ego is not in consciousness, which is utterly translucent, but in the world" (Sartre [1943] 1957:xii). For Sartre, consciousness has three stages, being-in-itself, being-for-itself, and being-for-others, which reflects a growing awareness. He argues that consciousness is intentional, it has a direction. In his attack on traditional psychology, Sartre is saying one must step back and ponder reality (there is a "power of withdrawal") because reality has a thoroughgoing impact on consciousness.

Consciousness is an awareness of oneself and the world. Furthermore, consciousness has depth, and as one moves through this space one's perception of oneself and the world changes. This does not automatically entail greater self-clarity. Movement through this "space-depth" is contingent on factors such as intelligence, curiosity, character, personality, experience, and chance; political-economic and cultural structures (class, race, gender, disability, age, sexual preference); and social institutions.

Evolution of consciousness depends on how one perceives and what questions one asks. What one concludes from the thousands of impulses and impressions one receives throughout life depends on, following Albert Einstein, where the observer is and how he or she observes. Take sunsets as an example. We "see" sunsets. But how we see a sunset depends on the weather (e.g., clouds), who we are with and our state of mind at the time, the vantage point (boat, beach, high-rise building), and so on. How we see a sunset is dependent on what we think a sunset is. For many, it is the descent of the sun below the perceived horizon. I can confirm this personally, having watched tourists jump into their tour bus immediately after the sun disappears. For others, the sunset continues until the sun's rays shine back against the darkening sky and produce a sublime radiance.

The point is that consciousness cannot be separated from the real world, from politics and culture. There is an important relationship between being and consciousness.[6] Social being informs consciousness, and consciousness informs being. There is a mutual interplay. Consciousness is not a container that ideas and experiences are poured into. Consciousness is a process of awareness that is influenced by social conditions, chance, and innate cognition.

People are sometimes described as not having consciousness. This is not so. Everyone has consciousness; it is just that for some, probably most, that consciousness is partially false. From childhood, people are constantly bombarded with the values of the dominant culture. These values reflect the "naturalness" of superiority and inferiority, dominance and subordination.

Power and Ideology

The greatest challenge in conceptualizing oppression of any kind is understanding how it is organized and how it is reproduced. It is relatively easy to outline general characteristics such as poverty, degradation, exclusion, and so on. But to answer these questions, we must examine the diffuse circuitry of power and ideology. This exercise is particularly difficult because power and ideology not only organize the way in which individuals experience politics, economics, and culture, they contradictorily obscure or illuminate why and how the dimensions of (disability) oppression are reproduced.

Oppression is a phenomenon of power in which relations between people and between groups are experienced in terms of domination and subordination, superiority and inferiority. At the center of this phenomenon is control. Those with power control; those without power lack control. Power presupposes political, economic, and social hierarchies, structured relations of groups of people, and a system or regime of power. This system, the existing power structure, encompasses the thousands of ways some groups and individuals impose control over others.

Power is diffuse, ambiguous, and complicated: "Power is more general and operates in a wider space than force; it includes much more, but is less dynamic. It is more ceremonious and even has a certain measure of patience. . . . [S]pace, hope, watchfulness and destructive intent, can be called the actual body of power, or, more simply, power itself" (Canetti [1962]1984:281). It is not simply a system of oppressors and oppressed. There are many kinds and experiences of power: employer/employee, men/women, dominant race/subordinated race, parent/child, principal/teacher, teacher/student, doctor/patient, to name some. Power more accurately should be considered power(s). These power relations are irreducible products of history. These histories of power(s) collectively make up the regime of power informing the manner and method of governing.

Power should not be confused with rule, however. A ruling class, historically forged by political and economic factors, governs. But other privileged groups and individuals have and exercise power. In the obscure vernacular of French philosophy, the relationship of power between those who are privileged and those who are not is *overdetermined* by class rule.[7]

There are many ways for significantly empowered classes and groups to exercise and maintain power. All regimes, regardless of political philosophy, have ruled through a combination of force and coercion, legitimation and consent. In the Western democracies and parts of the Third World, consent is prevalent and force seldom used. In many parts of the Third World, though, state-sponsored repression is common. The repressive practices of Third World dictatorships are well known and documented. In these countries there exists a pathology between military control and consent. People fear the government and the military because these institutions promote fear through constant harassment and repression.

The primary method through which power relations are reproduced is not physical—military force and state coercion—but metaphysical—people's consent to the existing power structure. This is certainly the case for the hundreds of millions of people with disabilities throughout the world. In chapter 5, I analyze the passive acquiescence of people with disabilities, individually and collectively, in the face of extraordinary lived oppression.

The passive acquiescence to oppression is partially based in what the British cultural historian Raymond Williams has called the "spiritual character" of power: "In particular, ideology needs to be studied to find out how it justifies and boosts the economic activities of particular classes; that is, the study of ideology enables us to study the intention of the articulate classes and the spiritual character of a particular class's rule" (1973:6). Williams is suggesting that the dominant classes and culture constantly and everywhere impress on people the naturalness or normality of their power and privilege. Williams, following Antonio Gramsci, called this process *hegemony*.[8] Hegemony is projected multidimensionally and multidirectionally. It is not projected like a motion picture projects images. The impulses and impressions, beliefs and values, standards and manners are projected more like sunlight. Hegemony is diffuse and appears everywhere as natural. It (re)enforces domination not only through the (armed) state but also throughout society: in families, churches, schools, the workplace, legal institutions, bureaucracy, and culture.

Schooling is a particularly notable example of this process because it cuts across so many boundaries and affects so many, including people with disabilities. If, as we are led to believe, the mission of schooling is teaching and learning, then the logical questions are, who gets to teach? what is taught? how do students learn? and, most important, why? First, let me suggest that schooling has two principal "political" functions. Its narrow purpose is to teach acquiescence to power structures operating in the educational arena. Its broad purpose is to teach acquiescence to the larger status quo, especially the discipline of its workforce.

How does this work? First teachers are trained. Then their training (knowledge) is certified and licensed. Education is "professionalized." Teachers become educational experts. Students sit in rows, all pointing toward this repository of knowledge. The teacher pours his or her knowledge into the students' "empty" heads didactically. There is little sharing of knowledge between the teacher and the student,[9] for the teacher has learned that the process is unidirectional. The curriculum itself is standardized and licensed by state education officials, often the same body that licenses teachers. Moreover, administrators are far removed from the classroom, their only regular contact with students being discipline. They allow little innovation and flexibility. Many administrators continue the same rules and programs for decades. Power comes from above. Everyone and everything in the schooling process is authorized. Students are, in Jürgen Habermas's term, *steered*. Numerous studies have shown that girls are treated differently from boys regardless of the teacher's gender. Students from some families are encouraged and others discouraged. Some, for example, students with disabilities, are segregated in different schools or classrooms.[10]

The latter point is particularly important for understanding the fundamental connections between ideology and power as they relate to disability. Students with disabilities, as soon as their disability is recognized by school officials, are placed on a separate track. They are immediately labeled by authorized (credentialed) professionals (who never themselves have experienced these labels) as LD, ED, EMH, and so on. The meaning and definition of the labels differ, but they all signify inferiority on their face. Furthermore, these students are constantly told what they can (potentially/expect to) do and what they cannot do from the very date of their labeling. This happens as a natural matter of course in the classroom.

All activists I interviewed who had a disability in grade school or high school told similar kinds of horror stories—detention and retention, threats and insults, physical and emotional abuse. In Chicago, I have colleagues and friends who were told they could not become teachers because they used wheelchairs; colleagues and friends who are deaf and went through twelve years of school without a single teacher who was proficient in sign language (they were told it was good for them because they should learn to read lips). I have visited segregated schools that required its personnel to wear white lab coats (to impress on the disabled students that they were first and foremost sickly). I know of a student art exhibition that was canceled because some drawings portrayed the students growing up to be doctors and other "unrealistic vocations."

It is possible to identify numerous ways that students with disabilities are controlled and taught their place: (1) labeling; (2) symbols (e.g., white lab coats, "Handicapped Room" signs); (3) structure (pull-out programs, segregated classrooms, "special" schools, inaccessible areas); (4) curricula especially designed for students with disabilities (behavior modification for emotionally disturbed kids, training skills without knowledge instruction for significantly mentally retarded students and students with autistic behavior) or having significant implications for these students; (5) testing and evaluation biased toward the functional needs of the dominant culture (Stanford-Binet and Wexler tests); (6) body language and disposition of school culture (teachers almost never look into the eyes of students with disabilities and practice even greater patterns of superiority and paternalism than they do with other students); and (7) discipline (physical restraints, isolation/time-out rooms with locked doors, use of Haldol and other sedatives).[11]

Special Education, like so many other reforms won by the popular struggle, has been transformed from a way to increase the probability that students with disabilities will get some kind of an education into a badge of inferiority and a rule-bound, bureaucratic process of separating and then warehousing millions of young people that the dominant culture has no need for. While this process is uneven, with a minority benefiting from true inclusionary practices, the overarching influences of race and class preclude any significant and meaningful equalization of educational opportunities.[12]

The sociopolitical implications of this process are clear to many disability rights activists.

Danilo Delfin: "Disability rights advocacy in Southeast Asia is very hard. Children are taught never to argue with their teacher. It is a long socialization process."

The Chicago educators and disability rights activists Carol Gill and Larry Voss interviewed twenty-one people who went through Special Education. Their survey respondents indicated that they believed that Special Education made them more passive and convinced them of their lot in life.[13]

We can begin to see the similarities between power and hegemony. Power, as Elias Canetti reminds us, is "more general and operates in a wider space than force," and hegemony, according to Raymond Williams, is "a whole body of practices and expectations, over the whole of living: our senses and assignments of energy, our shaping perceptions of ourselves and our world. It is a lived system of meaning and values . . . but a culture which has also to be seen as the lived dominance and subordination of particular classes" (Eagleton 1989:110). The meanings and values of society are defined by the powerful. Hegemony is omnipresent. It is embedded in the social fabric of life.

One of the ironies of hegemony is that the dominant culture's success in inculcating its contrived value system is contingent on the extent to which that worldview makes sense. On one level, and I will consider this in greater detail later, the legitimation of the dominant culture, marked by acquiescence and consent, is founded on real-world experiences. This is what Ellen Meiksins Wood means when she writes in *The Retreat from Class,*

What gives this political form its peculiar hegemonic power . . . is that the consent it commands from the dominated classes does not simply rest on their submission to an acknowledged ruling class or their acceptance of its right to rule. The parliamentary democratic state is a unique form of class rule because it casts doubt on the very existence of a ruling class. It does not achieve this by pure mystification. As always hegemony has two sides. It is not possible unless it is plausible. (1986:149)

We can recognize this clearly when it comes to disability. People with disabilities are usually seen as sick and pitiful, and in fact many became disabled through disease and most live in pitiful conditions. Furthermore, most people with disabilities are only noticed when they are being lifted up steps, or walk into an obstacle, or are being assisted across a street. Historically, most people with disabilities live apart from the rest of society. Most people do not regularly interact with people with disabilities in the classroom, at work, at the movies, and so on. Instead of curing the social conditions that cause disease and desperation, or removing the steps that necessitate assistance, the dominant culture explains the pitiful conditions people are forced to live in by creating a stratum or group of "naturally" pitiful individuals to conceal its pitiful status quo. The dominant culture turns reality on its head.

Today the mass media play the greatest role in what Noam Chomsky and Edward Herman (1988) called "manufacturing consent" through the use of filters that select and shape information. Indeed, its role in creating and promoting images has grown exponentially in recent times as its capacity to project images has grown. The philosopher Roger Gottlieb links the mass media's role in maintaining order to creating an "authorized reality." He echoes Wood's earlier point that this created truth must actually reflect certain aspects of reality:

In this complex sense, the media, like the state and the doctor, serve as authority figures. Their authority is derived from the compelling power of the images they produce—just as the authority of the medieval church derived from the size of its cathedrals. . . . And it is not foolishness or stupidity that leads us to take these images so seriously. It is the fact that real needs are manipulated into false hopes. Our needs for sexuality, love, community, an interesting life, family respect, and self-respect are transformed by the ubiquitous images of an unattainable reality into the sense that our sexuality, family, and personal lives are unreal. And it is this mechanism that sustains social authorities no longer believed to be legitimate. (1987:156, 159)

What images of disability are most prevalent in the mass media? Television shows depicting the helpless and angry cripple as a counterpoint to a poignant story about love or redemption. Tragic news stories about how drugs or violence have "ruined" someone's life by causing him or her to become disabled, or even worse, stories of the heroic person with a disability who has "miraculously," against all odds, become a successful person (whatever that means) and actually inched very close to being "normal" or at least to living a "normal" life. Most despicable are the telethons "for" *crippled* people, especially, poor, pathetic, crippled children. These telethons parade young children in front of the camera while celebrities like Jerry Lewis pander to people's goodwill and pity to get their money. In the United States surveys have shown that more people form attitudes about disabilities from telethons than from any other source.[14]

These images merge nicely with the language used to describe people with disabilities.[15] Consider, for example, "cripple," "invalid," "retard." In Zimbabwe, the term is *chirema,* which literally translates as "useless." In Brazil, the term is *pena,* which is slang for an affliction that comes as punishment. These terms are evidence of how people with disabilities are dehumanized. The process of assigning "meaning" through language, signs, and symbols is relentless and takes place most significantly in families, religious institutions, communities, and schools.

The dehumanization of people with disabilities through language (as just one obvious example) has a profound influence on consciousness. They, like other oppressed peoples, are constantly told by the dominant culture what they cannot do and what their place is in society. The fact that most oppressed people accept their place (read: oppression) is not hard to comprehend when we consider all the ideological powers at work. Their false consciousness has little to do with intelligence. It does have to do with two interactive and mutually dependent sources. The first is the capacity of ruling regimes to instill its values in the mass of people through double-speak, misdirection (blame the victim), naturalized inferiority, and legitimated authority. This is *hegemony*. The second is the psychological devastation people experience which creates self-pity and self-annihilation and makes self-awareness, awareness of peers, and awareness of their own humanity extremely difficult. This is *alienation*. Hegemony and alienation are two sides of the same phenomenon—ideological domination.[16]

In the case of disability, domination is organized and reproduced principally by a circuitry of power and ideology that constantly amplifies the normality of domination and compresses difference into classification norms (through symbols and categories) of superiority and normality against inferiority and abnormality.

CHAPTER 3

Political Economy and the World System

On one level a political economy of disability is easy to establish. That people with disabilities are powerless and poor is uncontestable. Every socioeconomic indicator says so.

As with political economy generally, the political economy of disability must be centrally concerned with class. That the vast majority of people with disabilities are poor, without many of the basic necessities to live a full and independent life, is primarily a function of class. This can be expressed from the reverse point of view as well: people with disabilities who have adequate financial resources have no problem procuring the most modern wheelchairs and prosthetics; rehabilitation and psychiatric services; and personal assistants, drivers, and readers. Although experienced differently, this is the case throughout the world.

Ed Roberts: "Those of us living in the United States and Europe have a safety net that doesn't exist in the Third World. I will say that even in the developed countries, how much ease we have with life mostly depends on our income and what resources our families have. For instance, I personally can treat inaccessibility or negative attitudes as annoyances, but for those without income or jobs, these become major problems that threaten their ability to get housing, personal assistants, transportation—namely, the necessities of life."

Maria da Comceição Caussat: "There is a big difference in Brazil between people who have money and people who don't. In fact, there are almost two cultural views about many things including disability based on these differences. The disabled with money suffer prejudices; but, unlike most people with disabilities in Brazil, they have access to quality wheelchairs, personal assistants, access to universities, cars, and so on. Poor disabled people do not have access to any of these things, including the most basic medical and rehabilitation services."

Rajendra Vyas: "The main issue for everyone in India is employment. It's an economic issue, a survival issue. Millions of people with disabilities are starving today in India. . . . I was lucky because my family was highly educated. There were medical men and women in my family for several generations. But for poor families I would have been a burden. Everything must be considered in economic terms when you are as poor as so many millions of people are in India. Eighty-nine percent of the blind children who come to Bombay to study are from rural areas that are so poor these children don't have access to education. All of the homeless blind living in institutions in Bombay are from the rural areas. Their families force them to leave."

The class position of people with disabilities (de)limits their possibilities in life. Will they have the opportunity go to school, or must they beg at an early age to survive? Will they live in safe and accommodating homes, or will they live in shantytowns, in nursing homes or asylums, or on the streets? The influence of class on the political economy of disability is not purely a matter of economic relation to production and the market. Class is a socially constructed relationship, informed by race, gender, disability, and social status.

Cornelio Nuñez Ordaz: "Almost everyone with a disability in Mexico is poor, so it might surprise you that there are divisions among us. The physically disabled have a greater chance and women have less chance for marriage or employment. The Indians, the ones who are indigenous, are the poorest. Many of us in Oaxaca have some Olmec heritage, but the truly indigenous are really poor."

Nuñez's comments are illuminating because they indicate how many intersecting influences inform aspects of political economy. Unfortunately, this nuanced class perspective has often been absent in political-economic analysis. Internationally, southern Africa offers the most obvious example where class is necessarily contingent on race. In the nations of Zimbabwe and South Africa class formation is the result of the colonization by Europeans who appropriated massive tracts of land and resources through the exercise of terror. White people with disabilities benefit from the high standards of living enjoyed by whites generally in the region. They often study abroad; have personal assistants, readers, and drivers; have specially equipped cars; and have access to modern technology (prosthetics, wheelchairs, computers). For the most part, the same options are not available to blacks. The contrast is striking.

Friday Mandla Mavuso: "I was disabled in 1974. I was shot by an African policeman for no apparent reason. . . . I was treated like a criminal, my family wasn't notified for a couple of days. Through a policeman who was a fellow soccer player, I was told that I was being framed and needed a lawyer. Three months later, I went to court. I was still in the hospital. I was really afraid of being assassinated at this point. At the hearing, I was charged with robbery, resisting arrest, and possession of a dangerous weapon. Finally, because of a lack of evidence and after a long time, I was discharged. I was very lucky and happy because it is almost impossible to be discharged in South Africa if you are black and have a different story than the white police. . . . I was hospitalized for four years. Two of those years, I had really bad pressure sores, and once those were cleared up, I had to wait an additional two years for a wheelchair even though the wheelchair was really an inferior one."

William Rowland: "I became blind at four through an accident. Through grade school and high school, I went to the school for the blind seventy-five miles from Capetown. Fortunately, I grew up in the most beautiful place in South Africa, Seapoint, which is a neighborhood in Capetown along the ocean. I loved the vivid scenery and beauty, and I remember coloring for hours at the ocean so I have very vivid memories of what I saw as a very young child. As I grew up, I became independent very quickly. It was easy for me to figure out how to walk without a cane and so on. Of course, when I became blind, I was unable to read the papers, so many of the social realities of South Africa were lost to me. So, I would often get very shocked when police would harass blacks and coloreds because of their race. . . . Everything in South Africa is determined by the history of apartheid. I can give you so many examples of this—from the violence to the poverty. If you are white you have every advantage in life, if you are black you have none. These advantages and disadvantages are legally sanctioned here. . . . After high school, I went to London to study as a physiotherapist. In London, I had to completely fend for myself. I had to find the subway, go shopping, do my own cleaning. I was in London for three years. The last two were some of the happiest times in my life. I got to go to plays, travel around, and I even played in a pub band one year before the Beatles were known. We used to play the music of Buddy Holly, the Shadows, and Cliff Richard. . . . [After] I received my Ph.D., I returned to South Africa."

The relationship of race to class is blurred in Asia and Latin America, although it is equally important. In Asia, ethnicity and nationality transcend race. The Vietnamese denigrate the Chinese; the Chinese do the same to Filipinos; Thais look down on Laotians; and almost everyone

hates the Japanese. The point here is that there are historical and contemporary political-economic reasons for these prejudices, just as in the
United States. This is not only the case when an oppressed group represents a small part of the population. For instance, blacks throughout
Latin America are superexploited and politically unrepresented (Romo
1995), even in a country like Brazil where 80 million to 90 million black
people live.

Maria Luiza Camêra: "You cannot understand why disabled people are
poorer in Bahia than any place else in Brazil unless you know that Bahia is
almost entirely black."

In Latin America, the color lines are more flexible. Much of the population is mixed-race. For example, *moreño* can mean "dark," "mixed
black," or even "Mediterranean," depending on where you are in the
region. Within this continuum, unlike in the United States or Europe,
economic position can influence one's racial status. However complex
the social construction of race is in Latin America, race continues to play
a critical role in class formation beyond the region's blurred black/
white dichotomies. There are tens of millions of indigenous Indians
who are the poorest people in the Central American highlands and the
Amazon. A million Japanese are extremely impoverished and ostracized
in São Paulo, Brazil's mega-metropolis. So class, sometimes in combination with other influences like race and gender and sometimes alone,
has a strong influence on the politics and economics of everyday lives
for millions of people with disabilities.

This is especially the case in underdeveloped regions, a central feature of the world political-economic system. The 1993 UN report, *Human Rights and Disabled Persons,* states that people with disabilities are
almost universally poor, degraded, and powerless. The report specifically
targets what they call the developing world, estimating there are 200
million people with disabilities living in conditions in which "poverty
and superstition prevent improvement in their condition."[1]

Underdevelopment and Disability

Nadine Gordimer begins her novel *July's People* with Antonio Gramsci's celebrated maxim about the dislocations of historical

transformation: "The old is dying and the new cannot be born; in the interregnum there arises a great diversity of morbid symptoms." The intended image of past, present, and future sets the stage for the ironic story of a white South African family's survival in a rural African village during revolution. It is a compelling appreciation of the complex and paradoxical conditions of underdevelopment in the Third World.

These conditions are immediately apparent in a visit to the Third World. For example, in Zimbabwe one finds a modern urban life in Harare and Bulawayo juxtaposed to huge plantations that export tobacco and coffee owned by a few white gentry and worked by millions of poor black subsistence farmers. All this within a nation-state that has a black president and governing party with an avowed nationalist and socialist history, now in the middle of an economic restructuring plan to satisfy the World Bank and the International Monetary Fund.

These morbid symptoms manifest themselves in strange ways for individuals trying to cope with political and economic crisis. Early in a trip to Zimbabwe in 1991, I had an experience that is illustrative. In a short conversation with a disabled street vendor in Bulawayo, the country's second-largest city, I found out he was anxious to make a sale because he needed money for a bus ticket to Johannesburg. I was amazed to find a black man in his early twenties who wanted to go to Johannesburg because he felt his economic opportunities were greater there (this was before apartheid was dismantled). I asked if he was serious. He took a moment, smiled, and said, "Well, I probably will have to stay in Soweto." A year later when I visited Johannesburg, I met many street vendors there from Malawi, Mozambique, and Namibia. Today, constellations of morbid political-economic and social conditions are readily observable throughout the Third World, a fact that all the disability activists I interviewed there remarked on. These conditions, contingencies of an evolving world system with a commanding capitalist center, can be summarized as follows:

- national economies in which key sectors (e.g., food, natural resources, banking, and transportation) are controlled by foreign companies and are predicated on export-oriented production and import substitution that has led to a crisis in both domestic agricultural and industrial production and in turn forced millions of poor people, mostly subsistence farmers and laborers, into the huge metropolitan areas (or more prosperous neighboring countries)[2] where extravagant wealth coexists with outrageous poverty;[3]

- local ruling elites that are repressive and brutal (military dictatorships are common), corrupt and incompetent, bombastic and arrogant, and good at stealing money and elections and terrorizing the citizenry;

- a much greater outflow of money and resources than that which flows in, spiraling foreign debts,[4] environmental despoliation, destruction of indigenous cultures and aping of foreign cultures.

It is within this context that the degree and scope of the problems of everyday life are filtered by the political economy of underdevelopment. As Bernard Magubane wrote in *The Political Economy of Race and Class in South Africa*, "The characteristic features of South Africa, as a social formation, reflect the interaction of internal developments, representing the historical process leading to the present structure of society and its classes plus the impact of the imperial factor, that is, the specific way in which the South Africa social formation relates to the world capitalist socioeconomic formation" ([1979] 1990:193–194). This allows us to understand why there is only one rehabilitation worker for every 300,000 blacks in South Africa or why there are 1,200 black physicians serving 25 million black people while 25,000 white doctors serve 5 million white people (*Washington Post*, May 24, 1994). When I asked activists what these political-economic conditions meant for people with disabilities, they spoke of conditions characterized by hunger, homelessness, isolation, degradation, violence and fear of violence, infanticide, and disease.

It is noteworthy that even in those parts of the Third World that have experienced significant economic growth, the lives of people with disabilities have remained precarious.

Danilo Delfin: "Although I live in Thailand because I work for Disabled Peoples' International, I am from the Philippines. In the Philippines, I believe people with disabilities are better off than in the rest of Southeast Asia because the country is more economically developed, which increases people's opportunities. Thailand is probably close. Nevertheless, the overriding issue for almost all people with disabilities in the entire region is just survival."

Thailand is one of the most economically developed countries in the Third World. It had a 10 to 15 percent growth rate over the last five years, and is a growing international trade power. Ironically, economic development in Thailand has had a simultaneous positive and negative effect on the country's disabled. On the positive side, modernization has meant that some of the backward ideas about disability are slowly changing. But while the boom has meant increased economic prosperity for a few, people with disabilities continue to exist outside these new opportunities. They are selling the same handicrafts or lottery tickets or drugs that they have always sold. Just as important, perhaps, development has created a contaminated, violent, and gridlocked urban environment that presents many obstacles for people with disabilities.

Narong Patibabsarakich: "Thailand is going through a lot of economic development so these primitive ideas [about disability] are not as strong. Beware of the development statistics, though. We have a 7 to 10 percent growth rate, but that is because of foreign investment. All the profits leave the country. For example, we are seeing many problems because of this growth, yes, problems. Bangkok has a lot of construction, but it is all for foreigners. The countryside has not changed, so people are moving to Bangkok to get jobs. But then we mainly have growth in the city slums. Also, one thousand cars are being sold in Bangkok every day so traffic is impossible. We have no roads to handle this volume. Because of this, car accidents are the number one reason for the increase in the number of people with disabilities."

So-called economic miracles have done little to cure the symptoms of underdevelopment for people with disabilities. Diseases like polio, eliminated elsewhere, still exist. Industrial accidents are more common in the less industrialized periphery than in the metropolis. Employment is unattainable. Millions of people with disabilities are starving, and many more are hungry. Underdevelopment has produced misery for hundreds of millions of people with disabilities. People with disabilities are the poorest, most isolated group in the poorest, most isolated places.

To underscore the consequences of this, consider the following:

- In most Third World countries, people with spinal cord injury (SCI) usually die within one or two years after becoming paralyzed, often from severe pressure sores or urinary tract infections. One hundred million people have disabilities caused by malnutrition. In some countries, 90 percent of children with disabilities die before they reach twenty and 90 percent of children with mental disabilities die before they reach age five (UNESCO 1995:9–14).

- In some African countries no education is available to children with disabilities. In India only 3 percent of boys with disabilities are educated (girls have almost no chance). Of the 2 million blind children in India today, only 15,000 receive any education—and only in urban areas (ibid., 14).

• There are more than 110 million land mines in sixty-four countries. There are 1.5 mines per person in Angola, a country where 120 people a month have become amputees every year since 1978. There are 10 million to 12 million mines in Afghanistan, or one for every two people. Egypt has 23 million land mines. The sole purpose of these weapons is disablement. These mines disable, both physically and psychologically, 500 people a week. Land mines had disabled more than 700,000 people through 1994. To remove all these land mines would cost $58 billion (ibid.).[5]

• In Asia, infants who are born with disabilities often end up in orphanages after being abandoned by their families, and a new law in China requires abortion and also sterilization to prevent the birth of children with disabilities.[6]

• Infanticide of girls and disabled boys is widely practiced throughout Africa and India,[7] and historically, children in India were purposely disabled to make them more effective beggars.[8]

• Although the people of Bangladesh live in extraordinary poverty, development experts at the Bangladesh Rural Development Programme see some "encouraging signs" for the rural poor, except for those in what these specialists call the "4th group," which is characterized as "an absence of good health." The report argues that downward mobility results from women-headed households or disability.

• In Brazil in the last ten years, 50,000 workers died in industrial accidents—six times as many as in the United States, which has 100 million more people. There are 3,000 reported accidents per day, and 500,000 Brazilian workers are disabled annually in work-related accidents (Williams 1989).

Modern Industrial Society and Disability

How does the political economy of disability oppression in modern industrial society compare to that in peripheral economic zones? The answer is, both very similar and very different, although it should be acknowledged that comparisons are complicated because distinctions, even demarcations, exist *within* these zones:

Rachel Hurst: In my perception there are three distinct sub-divisions [in Europe]. The first of these sub-divisions includes the Nordic countries and The Netherlands. The Nordic countries and The Netherlands have a long reputation of human rights and equality of opportunity for all their citizens. . . . Most Nordic countries have spent twice as much on social services than other countries. . . . In what I call the "colonial" countries [England, France, Germany, and Spain] the situation is somewhat different. The old traditions of class and elitism work against disabled people and they really do get to be the bottom of the pile. . . . In the under-developed countries [Portugal, Italy, Ireland, and Greece] there is the lack of any meaningful social provision. The majority of resources that are spent on disability go to segregated, professionally-run projects and programs. (Hurst 1995:529)

Returning to the question of comparison and recognizing the nuances, it is clear that people with disabilities are poor and powerless everywhere. I will use the United States as a barometer because of its dominant political-economic position and the notable progress people with disabilities have made there.[9] First, we can say that people with disabilities are typically unemployed (66 percent in the United States [NCD 1994]). Of those with disabilities that are defined as "less severe," 35.3 percent are unemployed; of those with severe disabilities, 87.7 percent are unemployed (USDOE 1992). The mean income of people with disabilities was $7,812 in 1992, and 42.3 percent of people with disabilities are officially categorized as "very poor," that is, have incomes below 125% of the poverty line. This is four times higher than that for people without disabilities (ibid.). Obvious social implications follow from these statistics. For example, adults with disabilities are four times more likely than those without disabilities to have less than a ninth-grade education (NCD 1994). It is also clear that people with disabilities are less politically influential and are taken less seriously as a political constituency than other oppressed peoples, for example, workers, women, African- Americans, Latinos, and gays and lesbians. Neither of these two comparisons implies that people with disabilities in the United States experience the degree of political-economic oppression that their counterparts in the Third World do. An annual income of $7,812 is extraordinary in the periphery. That 33 percent of all adults with disabilities under the age of sixty-five have jobs in the United States far surpasses the employment rate in any country in the Third World. While all national economies go through cycles of expansion and stagnation, pe-ripheral economies are locked in permanent crises even during periods of economic growth.

Although important political advances have been made in Third World nations, their scope and force are limited. The area of disability rights law is a case in point. Although many of the existing legal man-dates are often unenforced in the United States, there is the possibility of legal recourse. The U.S. Justice Department, state human rights agen-cies, and federal and state courts do examine instances of discrimination based on disabilities. While these efforts pale in comparison to what is needed (owing in large part to the marginal political influence of peo-ple with disabilities), there are few laws and no enforcement or legal re-course in Third World countries. As Rachel Hurst told me, Europe falls somewhere in between when it comes to disability rights.

An example of how economic forces affect people with disabilities dif-ferently concerns how and where disability has become a locus of profit. The extraordinary level of wealth in modern industrial societies coupled with the evolution of the welfare state has created an economic milieu wherein people with disabilities have acquired an exchange value. This has to do with the power of capital to control and dehumanize people, making them over into commodities that can be bought and sold.

Let me explain by backing up a little. Capital should not be recog-nized only as machinery or gross investment—what most economists define as the "man-made" factors of production. Rather, it should be considered as the relationships people have with each other in the broadly understood processes of production, exchange, and distribu-tion. This is the view Marx argued for in two thousand pages of *Capi-tal* and *Grundrisse*.[10] In *Beyond Capital,* Istvan Meszaros writes, "capi-tal is a historically created property relationship," and later, "a mode of control" (1995:13, 368).[11] Further, it is within each of these processes of production, distribution, and exchange that the law of value operates, a "law" that regulates the global exchange of commodities.[12] A neces-sary regulation as the development of the world economic system inex-orably transforms everything it touches into commodities. Most im-portant, the transformation of people into commodities hides their dehumanization and exploitation by other human beings; it becomes simply an economic fact of life.

Although people with disabilities are, at best, marginal to the work market, they experience commodification just as do people who work.

Whereas workers become commodities the moment they sell their labor (power) to others for a wage, people with disabilities become commodities the moment their disabling condition acquires an exchange value that a few people profit from.[13] This is what has happened in parts of the United States, Europe, and Japan.

Whole industries have been set up to rehabilitate, transport, educate, house, employ, and service people with disabilities in segregated, "special" settings. In the United States, paratransit companies, private schools, developers, and employment and service agencies are making millions of dollars in segregating people with disabilities. People with disabilities have not escaped the forces of capital. One example of this is the U.S. wheelchair industry. For thirty years, the monopoly of Everest-Jennings fettered the development of lightweight wheelchairs because of their need to maximize short-term profits. The company's biggest markets were insurance companies and hospitals—buyers that wanted wheelchairs that would last a long time without regard for whether they were user-friendly. While this prevented hundreds of thousands of people from getting around more easily, Everest-Jennings made millions.

Another example, one that touches more people, is the nursing home industry. Numerous studies have shown that living at home, in a house or an apartment, is better psychologically, more fulfilling, and cheaper than living in nursing homes.[14] Yet these institutions prosper when federal programs that foster living in the community are cut. There are also funding disincentives that the U.S. Congress, through Medicare and Medicaid, has created to ensure the profit bonanza of nursing homes. According to the activist disability journal *Mouth* (1995), there are 1.9 million people with disabilities living in nursing homes at an annual cost of $40,784, although it would cost only $9,692 a year to provide personal assistance services so the same people could live at home. Sixty-three percent of this cost is taxpayer funded. In 1992, 77,618 people with developmental disabilities (DD) lived in state-owned facilities at an average annual cost of $82,228, even though it would cost $27,649 for the most expensive support services to live at home. There are 150,257 people with mental illness living in tax-funded asylums at an average annual cost of $58,569. Another 19,553 disabled veterans also live in institutions, costing the Veterans Administration a whopping $75,641 per person.[15] It is illogical that a government would want to pay more for less. It is illogical until one studies the amount of money spent by the nursing home lobby. Nursing homes are a growth industry that many wealthy people, including politicians, have wisely invested in. The scam is simple: get taxpayers to fund billions of dollars to these institutions which a few investors divide up.

The idea that nursing homes are compassionate institutions or necessary resting places has lost much of its appeal recently, but the barrier to defunding them is built on a paternalism that eschews human dignity. As we have seen with public housing programs in the United States, the tendency is to warehouse (surplus) people in concentrated sites. This too has been the history with elderly people and people with disabilities in nursing homes. These institutions then can serve as a mechanism of social control and, at the same time, make some people wealthy.

We do have better models and evidence of the superiority of these alternative models to nursing homes and other institutionalized living arrangements. People with severe disabilities who are living at home with personal assistance have demonstrated that living in an environment they control is far superior to institutionalized care. But according to the World Institute on Disability, "9.6 million people with disabilities live in the U.S. who need help with daily activities like washing, dressing and household chores. Less than 2 million receive paid assistance. Most rely on family and friends" (WID 1995). All of the 7.6 million people dependent on family or friends for personal assistance are thus vulnerable to future institutionalization.

In *The Disability Business,* Gary Albrecht examines the billions of dollars spent on "rehabilitation." Albrecht, in the course of examining a wide range of institutions and services from hospitals and rehabilitation agencies to charities and insurance companies, points out that nursing homes collect 8.4 percent of the $647 billion (1988 dollars) spent on national health in the United States. Who owns them? Primarily large corporations, among them, Humana, Hospital Corporation of America (Beverly Enterprises), and Summit Health Ltd. (Albrecht 1992:137–149). The micro political economy of disability is big business. These are not questions of preference or mistaken policies. These are questions of the political economy of disability.

Beyond Political Economy and Class Analysis?

This chapter has been necessarily observational. The definitive political economy of disability has yet to be written. I hope to have shown, however, that political-economic structures and systems are fundamentally part of the phenomenon of disability oppression. Data sets and analyses of how and where the exploitation and commodification of people with disabilities take place will not change the simple fact that they are poor and powerless. In addition, what seems like a reasonable proposition to me—the centrality of class in contemporary relations of power and domination—is widely criticized as anachronistic and obsolete. Through a variety of structural and ideological changes, class analysis has become an unsuspecting relic of an increasingly fragmented world.

There is, of course, some justification for this view. Disability as a social category fragments class because of its heterogeneous class origins and nonclass identity. Furthermore, there has been a change in the way in which capital accumulation takes place—the transition from Fordism to flexible accumulation—and the way in which power relations are ideologically reinforced—the increased capacity and power of advertising and the media.[16] In the final analysis, though, the objection to class seems like a repetition of the age-old denial of class by traditional sociology and bourgeois economic theory or, more to the point, the disillusioned defeatism of leftist academicians more than any fundamental shift in the motor force of economic and political necessity. For the last five hundred years the need to accumulate and the need to control remain unchanged. The inexorable and remorseless drive for profit maximization is no more or less an option today than it was twenty or fifty years ago. In fact, while today the world political-economic system is more fluid than ever, it is also more integrated than ever. The process of globalization has replaced the internationalization of capital in that foreign capital not only flows across national borders along fiber-optic computer channels in microseconds, it functionally controls internationally dispersed economic activities. The global political economy will, I believe, increase, not decrease, the importance of class in the lives of people with disabilities, even those in remote areas.

As Nancy Hartsock has pointed out, political economy is not only important in understanding the dynamics of these developments, it provides a context for understanding other crucial influences on everyday lives: "I would still insist that we not give up the claim that material life [class position, in Marxist theory] not only structures but sets limits on the understanding of social relations, and that in systems of domination, the vision available to the rulers will be both partial and will reverse the real orders of things" (1990:172). For without political economy, culture, ideology, and consciousness often lose their coherence or are obscured. This is not to say that the relationships among them are unidirectional—from political economy to everything else. They are multidirectional and mutually informing. Political-economic, cultural, family, gender, racial, ideological, religious, and legal structures are all interdependent. The political-economic structure, though, tends to position people, groups, belief systems, social structures, and ideologies in relation to each other. In terms of oppression, it is both a producer and product of systems of domination and subordination and of ideologies of superiority and inferiority.

CHAPTER 4

Culture(s) and Belief Systems

Culture exerts a profound influence on the way in which people think and what they think. An individual's beliefs—whether religious, aesthetic, moral/ethical, political, or philosophical—produce his or her worldview. A worldview not only imparts meaning, it positions beliefs in relation to rituals, habits, laws, grammar, facial expressions, body image, sex and sexuality, artifacts, games, and so on. Culture is "the realm of the symbolic—that amorphous web of values, beliefs, assumptions and ideals that we internalize by being members of certain groups in a certain place at a certain time. It is within the realm we call culture that we get our bearings in life; it is there that we ingest the notions of what is good, bad, just, natural, desirable, and possible" (NACLA 1994:15). The impression of culture on beliefs and mythology, traditions and rituals, institutions and doctrines, has individual and social implications. First, culture is a milieu and medium of domination and subordination. The beliefs, ideas, and values of society at large not only reflect the dominant culture, they help to reproduce it. Second, beliefs and the attitudes they spawn are not solely determined by religious convictions or education or class or words, symbols, and expressions, or even the mass media. They are informed by the interplay of all these.

Beliefs and attitudes about disability are individually experienced but socially constituted. They are, with few exceptions, pejorative. They are paternalistic and often sadistic and hypocritical. When blatantly pejorative attitudes are not held, people with disabilities often experience a paradoxical set of "sympathetic" notions like the courageous or noble individual. Attitudes such as "I couldn't adjust to such a life, he must

51

be so strong" or "She has overcome so much to be successful" derive from and feed the same beliefs as pity, contempt, or shame. That is, if a person with a disability is "successful," or seems to have a good life, he or she is seen as brave and courageous or special or brilliant. Given the intrinsic abnormality or awfulness of disability, anyone living a "normal" or ordinary life must be extraordinary.

Attitudes can be paradoxical in other ways as well. In a few cultures such as the Yoruba in Nigeria and the Hubeer in Somalia disability may carry secondary deity status (even when the cause of disability is looked on as a tragedy). As the art historian Ulli Beier pointed out more than two decades ago, "The creation story of the Yorubas says that Obatala created human beings out of clay. When he had finished molding their forms, he would give them to Olorum, who would blow life into them. One day, however, Obatala went drinking. That day he created albinos, cripples, and blind people. In memory of that day, the worshippers of the Orisa [deity] are forbidden to drink palm wine; and afflicted people are considered to be especially sacred to the god and they are given positions of some importance in his shrines" (1969:12).[1]

A General Formulation of Attitudes toward Disability

The problem of disabled persons in Brazil is closely related to the history and overall situation of all Brazilian people. The paternalistic approach of the Brazilian elite has been responsible for the notion that (1) there are no prejudices against minorities and other social groups and (2) these groups are well integrated in the larger society.

Program of the Movement for the Rights of Disabled Persons (Brazil)

Periodically, relatives would come to my family's house and they would intend to ask how are you, how are you managing, but they would use a vernacular that really felt like I had just got out of intensive care, like I was dying, like I was sick.

Ranga Mupindu, executive director of the National Council of Disabled Persons of Zimbabwe

Paternalism lies at the center of the oppression of people with disabilities. Paternalism starts with the notion of superiority: We must and can take control of these "subjects" in spite of themselves, in spite of their individual will, or culture and tradition, or their sovereignty. The savages need to be civilized (for their own good). The cripples need to be cared for (for their own good). The pagans need to be saved (for their own good). Paternalism is often subtle in that it casts the oppressor as benign, as protector. The relation between ideology and power is expressed as natural to justify relations of oppression. In *Roll, Jordan Roll,* possibly the best-known exposition of paternalism, Eugene Genovese writes,

The Old South, black and white, created a historically unique kind of paternalist society. . . . Southern paternalism, like every other kind of paternalism, had little to do with Ole Massa's ostensible benevolence, kindness, and good cheer. It grew out of the necessity to discipline and morally justify a system of exploitation. . . . For the slaveholders, paternalism represented an attempt to overcome the fundamental contradiction in slavery: the impossibility of the slaves ever becoming the things they were supposed to be. Paternalism defined the involuntary labor of the slaves as a legitimate return to their masters for protection and direction. (1976:4–5)

Paternalism often must transform its subjects into children or people with childlike qualities. This is the most salient aspect of paternalism as it concerns disability. Paternalism is experienced as the bystander grabs the arm of a blind person and, without asking, "helps" the person across the street. This happens for wheelchair users as well. It is the experience of the waiter asking a companion of a person with a disability, "What does she want to eat?" It is the institutionalization of people against their wishes. It is the child taught only handicrafts, or the charity pleading for money to help cute crippled kids. It is these and a thousand other examples of everyday life. It is most of all, however, the assumption that people with disabilities are intrinsically inferior and unable to take responsibility for their own lives.

This kind of paternalism is also experienced by women. Henrik Ibsen captured it in *A Doll's House.* Ibsen's Nora was one of the first literary characters to challenge the paternalism of male supremacy through establishing a counterimage of the helpless, childlike woman:

Nora: During eight whole years, and more—ever since the first day we met—we have never exchanged one serious word about serious things.

Helmut: Was I always to trouble you with the cares you could not help me bear?

Nora: I am not talking about cares. I say that we have never yet set our-selves seriously to get to the bottom of anything.

Helmut: Why, my dearest Nora, what have you to do with serious things?

Nora: There you have it! You have never understood me. I have had great injustice done me, Torvald; first by father, then by you. (Quoted in Schneir 1972:182)

The myth of women as helpless or weak has always been an ideolog-ical foil for women's oppression, a paternalism, as Mary Wollstonecraft wrote a hundred years before Ibsen, that "degrade[s] one half of the hu-man species, and render[s] women pleasing at the expense of every solid virtue" (ibid., 7). In contrast to the paternalism of slavery, which con-signed responsibilities to the slaves in the form of labor, paternalism to-ward women and people with disabilities denies the intrinsic capacity for or interest in managing responsibilities.[2]

Paternalism, like other dominant ideologies, is built on partial expe-rience. As Ellen Meiksins Wood and Perry Anderson have argued, no idea—no matter how ardently promoted by the dominant ideology—can take hold unless it partially reflects the real experiences of people (Wood 1986:149). This has been particularly powerful in the case of people with disabilities because until very recently they have not con-tested the backward ideas of the dominant culture by demanding recog-nition, respect, and responsibility. People with disabilities may have in-dividually resisted the degradation of paternalism, but they have never done so collectively.

Moreover, many belief systems combine with paternalism to cast dis-ability as physically or metaphysically tainted. This is most prominent in the least developed areas of the Third World, but it exists everywhere. Most important, people with disabilities are conceived, in the first place, as in-ferior and as the embodiment of bad luck, misfortune, or religious pun-ishment. The disability itself primarily informs the conception most people have about individuals with disabilities. Their humanity is stripped away and the person is obliterated, only to be left with the condition—dis-ability. This is why Irving Zola insisted that people with disabilities should never allow themselves to be described by a noun—"the blind," "the deaf," "the disabled." "No matter what label is used," he writes, "it cannot help but equate the person totally with his/her disability" (1984:2).

Although feminists have provided a penetrating and effective critique of paternalism, it is still a powerful ideological system. I would argue that the phenomenology of disability oppression parallels that of women's oppression based on our similar experiences with paternalism. In the interviews I conducted, pity and shame, emotions that women have experienced, were the two most commonly identified attitudes toward disability.

Shame and pity can be considered the two sides of paternalism that are most significant in the formation of attitudes about disability. Shame looks in, pity looks upon. In *Femininity and Domination*, Sandra Bartky writes, "Shame can be characterized in a preliminary way as a species of psychic distress occasioned by a self or a state of the self apprehended as inferior, defective, or in some way diminished" (1990:85). Shame takes place in relation to others. That is, people with disabilities or their family members or friends feel shame when they themselves relate to disability in front of others, or in society. Bartky points this out by quoting Sartre: shame is "in its primary structure shame before somebody" (ibid.). Pity, like its source, paternalism, presupposes superiority. It is projected onto people. People with disabilities are primarily *subjects* of pity. The lives of people with disabilities are (considered) less, because their bodies and minds are (considered) less. To pity is to actually look at and feel bad for them. Pity is an emotion that is rooted in sight. It does not take any other factors into account. A person who cannot see or is using a wheelchair for mobility may be a happy, prosperous, well-adjusted person, but most people encountering him or her immediately feel pity.

Three Progenitors of Attitudes toward Disability

Comprehending why attitudes toward disability are universally negative requires tracing their genealogy into the many sociocultural realms that have crucial importance in socialization. In this section, I will concentrate on three of these: body/image, religion, and language. These, in their own right and in combination with other influences, predominantly inform attitudes about disability for the vast majority of the world's people.

THE BODY: WHERE SCIENCE AND IMAGE MEET

*Captive. Sabotaged by my own body. I sit here seething,
glaring at this pillowy snowfall, caught in a web of my dream,
the taste of powerlessness it leaves behind. In Maine I was*

fighting forces much too great for me: wind, snow, stunning
cold, and of course, loneliness. It was hopeless and I knew it,
but I persisted, doomed and so absorbed in the minutiae of the
struggle that I forgot hopelessness. (Self-reliance, ha.) This
time the enemy is me, the crumbling temple of my cancerous
body, stitched together like a Raggedy Ann doll.

Protagonist in Jean Stewart's *The Body's Memory*

Historically, disability has been considered a priori a medical condition and people with disabilities, sick. This has nothing to do with disease per se but with a medical category. If people with disabilities are first a category of medicine, then by definition we are intrinsically ill, with infirm bodies and minds. People with disabilities are often set apart and identified by their "bodies" and their appearance. The fusion of science (medicalization) and body (image) is a powerful constraint.

No subject is more hotly debated by academics today than "the body." This has happened in the wake of the ascendancy of poststructuralism, especially the theories of Michel Foucault. Foucault was interested in power. As he reduced his scope of inquiry, he quickly got to the body: "Indeed I wonder whether, before one poses the question of ideology, it wouldn't be more materialist to study first the question of the body and the effects of power on it" (Foucault 1980:58). Questions about the body are immensely important to the examination of attitudes toward disability. As Rosemarie Garland Thomson writes, "Our traditional account of disability casts it as a problem located in bodies rather than a problem located in the interaction between bodies and the environment in which they are situated" (1995:16).

Cultures impart meaning through the ways in which characteristics of the body are given value or status. John Thompson, in *Ideology and Modern Culture,* termed this the "process of valorization" (1990:145). The facial scar in the Americas is considered a deformation, but for the Dahomey in Africa it is a badge of honor. Most cultures consider fat unattractive, but it is beautiful in Polynesia. Even among cultures that consider fat unattractive, some are influenced more than others by what Bartky called "the tyranny of slender" (1990:73). In many Asian cultures, for example, the body is only one of many attributes informing attractiveness. In Latin America or North America, it is the essential factor. Foucault provides an interesting—but limited—vantage point from which to appreciate the historical medicalization of disability.[3] Foucault's paradigm, which situates the body as the only verifiable "truth" or site of oppression, contradicts the political thrust of the disability rights movement, which posits that disability is an oppressed social condition. This latter view is also advanced by the anthropologist Terence Turner in his critique of poststructuralism: "The current fetishism of the body in cultural theory must be accounted for, not as a straightforward case of consciousness-raising by history, but rather as an instance of ideological reification of precisely the kind that many leading proponents of contemporary body theory proclaim themselves, in the name of the body, to have transcended" (1995:170). The point that Turner makes so well is that the body, like culture generally, is informed by historical and social processes—most important, practical activity. The oppression of individual disabled bodies is not the basis for the oppression of people with disabilities, it is the oppression of people collectively that is the basis for the oppression of their bodies.

Recently there have been a number of important inquiries into and descriptions of embodiment and disability. These range from the disability rights activist Jean Stewart's novel *The Body's Memory* to the anthropologist Robert Murphy's historiography *The Body Silent* to Gelya Frank's ethnography "On Embodiment." Each of these treats the disabled body as central. How they treat it varies greatly. Kate, Jean Stewart's protagonist, in a series of letters and poems, evolves an awareness of her disabled body as an oppressed body. Stewart's personal experience with disability is informed by her participation in the disability rights movement. Murphy's orientation is markedly different because of his lack of involvement with the DRM. His isolation is evident in a defeatism that senses disability as a unidirectional assault on identity and a necessary dislocation or separation from family and community. Without questioning the veracity of Murphy's own experience with disability, his extension of this to a generality is unsatisfactory. On a personal level Murphy misses what is (potentially) gained from disability in terms of identity, insight, and comradeship. Gelya Frank takes an observational approach in her treatment of the disabled body. Her examination of Diane DeVries's growing self-consciousness is an important contribution to understanding how women with disabilities develop positive self-images in spite of an array of reactionary, body-centered ideas.

In the practical bodily activities of everyday life, disability presents real and often poorly understood limitations. These limitations, whether physical, sensory, or cognitive, are impulses for the production, transmission, and reception of images, meanings, rituals, and folklore in particular cultures. Popular culture has become infatuated with body imagery. Bodies have become commodities that sell everything from beer to black bean dip. Bodies that sell are beautiful ones, and beauty is defined by how the dominant culture produces and markets images. Recently this has been at the service of sex. Many futurists contend that soon there will be little that distinguishes body beautiful from sex itself.[4]

This is an epiphenomenon of disability oppression. The future importance of body and sexual imagery, especially where they intersect, will no doubt increasingly have an impact on people with disabilities. That the selling of the body beautiful and its nexus to sex has withstood trenchant criticism from feminism should not be lost on the DRM (Galler 1984; hooks 1992; Morrison 1970; Wolf 1991). As the mass culture increasingly embraces these images as their own, people will become increasingly defined by them. The ramifications are especially bad for women with disabilities.

Rosangela Berman Bieler: "In spite of the similar discrimination disabled men and women face, there is a point where they differ: in sexuality and affection. Latin countries like Brazil have machoist aesthetic values that make a woman with a perfect body the 'ideal' type. This notion, which is exhaustively exploited by the media, generates an enormous gap between women and men, disabled or not."

The cruel treatment of women with disabilities is rooted, in many cultures, in the dehumanization of those women based in part on their dual body status—as women and as women with disabilities. Some women I interviewed reported they had been raised by their families to become good housekeepers but never to become sexually active women. Some said they never had full-size mirrors at home which permitted a view of their bodies as they grew up. One woman said as a child she frequently was lectured, "When your brothers marry, you'll live with them and help take care of their children." Moreover, everyday bodily issues such as appearance, body language, facial expressions, and posture are almost universally neglected, making these issues, especially sexuality, extremely problematic.

The implications of the present image of the disabled body—its abnormality and its ugliness—are clear. This image leads inevitably to the notion that people with disabilities are asexual. This is a powerful myth, because it is not only a product of the medicalization of disability, it is steeped in and reinforces the paternalism that consigns people with disabilities to a permanent status as children.

Maria Paula Teperino: "When I was married many people asked our maid if she could hear whether we had sex. Everyone on the street would ask me, for example, if we could have a baby. That was the first question many people thought about."

Cornelio Nuñez Ordaz: "I got married in 1978 when I was twenty-five. I met my wife on the way to the Rehab Center. First we were friends and then we got married. It was very difficult for her to be with me because her friends thought she shouldn't date a disabled man, they assumed we wouldn't or couldn't have sex, I'm not sure. During my wife's first pregnancy a lot of family and friends told us they were afraid that the child would be born with a disability."

The issue of sexuality for people with disabilities brings into relief the relationship between gender and disability mythology. Here the influences of sexuality, sexism, paternalism, and sexual repression meet, creating all sorts of ironies.

Maria Paula Teperino: "There is a cult of the body in Brazil. We call it *culto ao corpo.* You really need beautiful legs and bottoms in our culture. Machismo is very strong, and it affects the way many men think of women. Because of its prevalence, machismo leads many men to believe that a disabled woman can't satisfy him. Many even believe that disabled women cannot have children. Sons are considered necessary by Brazilians. . . . Even though my mother always encouraged me to dress well and look pretty [as I grew up], I believe she never thought I would get married. It's strange because I know she believed I would lead an intellectual and independent life, but the issue of dating and sexuality never was discussed. This was a double message and confusing, but looking back on it, I shouldn't be surprised. The myths and stereotypes about disability and sexuality based in our macho culture taught her these ideas."

Many activists believe that the men most influenced by the macho worldview have been the most condemned by it after their disability.

Federico Fleischmann: "If a man in Mexico has an accident like you, let's say at the age of forty, that's the end. I don't know one that beats this kind of problem. They stay home, and they think they are half a man. It's very difficult because of our culture in which the macho image is very strong. If you cannot play soccer any more, life has no value. Mexican culture, machismo, has a very negative effect on a man becoming disabled."

These notions extend far beyond Latin America.

Lizzie Mamvura: "In Zimbabwe, the attitudes toward disabled women are very backward. For example, in my village, but also in Bulawayo, I was told many times that no man would want me as a woman because I had a disability. In fact, there was a strange man who always said I was his wife and this was very annoying. Finally, after a lot of effort, I built up my nerve and told him to stop this practice. He said no one would want me so he was doing me a favor. I stood up to him, and from then on I felt a lot stronger. I felt the power of talking for myself. The women's project I coordinate has this issue as a major goal. That is, to hold meetings and workshops that train leaders and others to be assertive. To speak up, to articulate our rights—the right to work, to get married, have kids. Unfortunately, we are a small minority. The biggest problem is that it's very difficult for disabled women to get married and to find a job. Even if a man is interested in marriage, his parents wouldn't allow it. They believe that having their son marry a disabled woman would bring misfortune or bad luck to the family. Also, there is widespread unemployment and Zimbabwean culture expects women to stay in their village. It is doubly bad for a disabled woman because she is shut off by people in the village and even her family."

Fadila Lagadien: "I became involved in women's issues because of sexuality issues more than discrimination. Through the disability movement, I fight for human rights because women with disabilities are told not to have children, that we are asexual, and often there is forced sterilization. In South Africa, families don't educate or support the education of disabled women because of the attitude that no man will pay a *bola* [dowry] for a disabled woman."

The similarities in Western culture should not be overlooked. In "Daughters with Disabilities," Harilyn Rousso writes, "There is a myth in our society that disabled people are asexual. . . . Because so much of female sexuality has focused on physical appearance, disabled women are particularly likely to be misperceived as asexual" (1988:140). As a practical matter, the presumption that disability is equated with asexuality has meant that people with disabilities are not socially and emotionally prepared to experience their own sexuality. Rousso again:

Parental difficulty in recognizing and affirming the social and sexual potential of disabled daughters can be understood in terms of the individual dynamics of the parents and family, and in terms of broader societal values. For mothers in particular, affirmation of sexual potential and womanhood may require the mother's ability to see herself in her daughter and to be able to identify with her. As a result of their own dynamics and history, for some mothers the daughter's disability may loom too large and make the daughter seem too disparate; the mother may then have difficulty identifying and seek to keep her distance. For example, the disability may remind the mother of her own feelings of imperfection, and she may be reluctant to acknowl-

edge that part of herself. Or, having a disabled child may seem like punishment for wrongdoing, a source of guilt safer dealt with from afar. Fathers
also play an important role in the confirmation of a female child's heterosexuality. For fathers to affirm their daughter's heterosexuality, they must
be able to see in their daughters the potential to become the kind of woman
they could choose as a mate. Again, as a result of feelings of inadequacy,
guilt, or other dynamics, the father may have difficulty seeing his daughter
in this light. (Ibid., 152–153)

Disability itself is the embodiment of repulsive images of *the body*, certainly a body no one would want to have sex with. The paternalistic idea
that people with disabilities are asexual contributes to the idea that they
are less human, invalid or less valid. If one is innately asexual, one has
something less to give and to be.

   This imaged meaning of the disabled body is refined and reinforced
by many ideological agents, most important, the mass media. The media's relentless production of images, in large part processed and
screened through its depiction of sexuality, family life, and personal lives,
is created, packaged, and marketed with assumptions about the body's
importance. In response to this, a number of activist North American
and European academics in the DRM have begun their own analyses
and critiques. Important work has been done, for example, by Harlan
Hahn (1989) and Paul Longmore (1987). Longmore, one of North
America's best-known writers on disability imaging, sums up the mass
media's projection of disability: "The most prevalent image in films and
especially in television during the past several decades has been the maladjusted disabled person. These stories involve characters with physical
or sensory, rather than mental handicaps. The plots follow a consistent
pattern: The disabled central characters are bitter and self-pitying because, however long they are disabled, they have never adjusted to their
handicaps, and never accepted themselves as they are" (1987:70). There
are, of course, maladjusted people with disabilities who are bitter or self-
pitying, but the ideological implications of these images go much deeper.
They suggest that any "problem" that might develop for a person with
a disability is individually based, simultaneously obliterating oppression
and any socially produced barriers. Many activists from the Third World
echo Longmore's assessment of the U.S. media.

Maria Paula Teperino: "Our culture is shaped so much in Brazil by the media. The media forces the picture that disabled people are not able to do
certain things like have sex and be happy. An example was the polio and

virus vaccination campaigns in the past. Brazil eliminated these about ten to twelve years ago. But in the television propaganda that was used to encourage people to get the vaccine, the message always was, until about four years ago, you had better get these shots or you will get the disease, become disabled, and your life will be ruined because you will be sick for the rest of it. . . . Many of the angry characters in our soap operas use wheelchairs. When they stop being mean, they're cured of their disability. Disability, then, is in your head. A lot of the disabled on the TV soaps turn out not to have a disability, it was only in their heads. So when they are feeling better and are happy, then they become cured of their disability."

The dominant cultures in the world produce images of normality and abnormality, of beauty and ugliness, of superiority and inferiority. These images are projected by their producers to influence opinions and preferences. The sick/deformed body is stuck at the intersection where science and image meet.

GOD, BUDDHA, AND DEAD ANCESTORS

Cambodia [Kampuchea] is the worst off. It's the poorest, and their attitudes toward us are the worst. Their Buddhism says that if you lack some body function, you lack perfection, you are tainted.

Danilo Delfin, Southeast Asia regional development
officer, Disabled Peoples' International

In 1993 I sat in the conference room of the largest social service agency in Thailand. In the room were leaders of all the disability groups in the country that are consumer controlled. All disabilities were well represented. The main topic was the relationship between attitudes toward disability and the barriers to social progress. After an hour or so everyone had clearly articulated the need to change attitudes that defined disability as pitiful, sad, sick, a burden, something bad. After a break I changed directions a bit and asked people to talk about their religious beliefs. Of the eleven people present, all but one were Buddhists. This was to be expected, as 97 percent of Thais are Buddhists. Many described the Buddhist notion of reincarnation. They affirmed the reason that people tried to live a good spiritual life was to avoid having a difficult existence in their next life.

I asked the ten Buddhists if they believed they had a disability because of something bad they had done in a previous life. All but one raised their hands. I then asked if they did not see a contradiction between this belief and their collective interest in changing society's attitudes about disability. They looked at each other in dismay. The room became quiet. They realized their religious beliefs conflicted with their political and social beliefs.

This example illustrates the dilemma that disability rights activists who are religious face. They must reject a fundamental aspect of their belief or deny its conservative character. Reincarnation represents only one of the many socioreligious myths that influence the notion of disability. Others hold that disability comes from the gods or ancestral spirits or witches, from sin or lack of ancestor homage. Given different cultures, the responses to these beliefs may range from annoyance to a social sanction that isolates or even vilifies people. For example, witchcraft is a very powerful force in rural Africa and among some African-based religious sects of Latin America, especially Brazil and the Caribbean.

Joshua Malinga: "Now in Africa we have very backward ideas about disability connected to witchcraft and to life as an oppressed people historically."

Alexander Phiri: "In our culture, disability is looked at as shameful not just for the disabled person but for the family. This is connected to witchcraft, to some notions that somehow the ancestors are upset because the family is not acting in the traditional way or honoring them enough. The traditional religious churches do not even attempt to change these ideas because they are afraid of losing members."

Ranga Mupindu: "People who were superstitious believed evil spirits had cursed me."

In Africa, ancestral spirits are widely respected. Many Africans engage *sangomos* (witch-doctors) to help appease these spirits (*lidlotis* in Swazi). Sangomos exist in other places, with some similar and dissimilar roles and tasks, for example, *curanderos* and *brujos* in Mexico and *dukens* in Indonesia. Shamans, sorcerers, prophets—all play influential roles in the way their communities perceive and relate to many things, including disability. These people are often thought of as healers. Because disability is perceived as a medical condition, people with disabilities often fall within the purview of these curers. Their influence, although waning under the advance of science and Western culture, is strongest in rural areas.[5]

Religion and spirituality interact with disability in two major ways. First, religion links the origin of disability to sin, witchcraft, (black) magic, a past grievance, bad karma,[6] lack of ancestor worship, and so on.

Disability, then, is equated with something negative, even evil. Second, religion, and especially spirituality, locates progress in the realm of otherness such as heaven or nirvana, and the vehicle to it is individual purity, acceptance, prayers, alms. "In Palau, the question of what caused a disability is of primary importance—not the medical cause, but the spiritual cause. All disabilities are believed to be caused by some failure on the part of someone to follow a tradition, fulfill a responsibility, appease an ancestor" (Mallory 1992:14).

Rosangela Berman Bieler: "Brazilians look at people with disabilities as superheroes or as pitiful. Church is immensely important to these attitudes. The biggest Catholic church in the world is here. But Catholicism is declining and evangelism is growing in our country. The Catholic church fights with African religious traditions, whereas the evangelicals don't. The evangelicals stress that God will take the devil from your body, which for me means that I'll be able to walk. These people are very obnoxious. Every day, somebody will stop me and tell me I should find God and be happy. I tell them I'm already happy. They say no one can be happy in a wheelchair. I just laugh at them. While the Catholic church is backward in many ways because it promotes pity, it is not nearly as bad as these evangelicals who think the devil is inside us."

While religion hosts a panoply of reactionary ideas about disability, the institutional church may be worse. Throughout the world, the role of the church has been tied historically to colonial wealth and support of the existing social order. This has been the case with the Catholic church in concert with Spanish and Portuguese colonialism in the Americas, the northern European colonization of Africa in the guise of its messianic role to "civilize" that continent, or British hegemony and the Church of England in Asia.

One million Indians died in the mines of Peru (Galeano 1985:172, 224) and the Catholic church uttered not a word. Half a million Indonesians died at the hands of the Suharto regime in the late 1960s, and Moslems turned inward. Thousands starve each day in India, and the Hindu religion emphasizes individual contemplation. If one wants change, any kind of change, support cannot be found within the traditional religious institutions (with the exception of the marginally influential segment of the Catholic church that espouses liberation theology). They represent and reflect the status quo, both past and present. Judy Kugelmass, in her investigation of the family's adaptation to mental disability in West Java, points out the barriers to progress posed by a fusion of political and religious mythology:

A Javanese or Sudanese person will rarely answer a direct question with a direct, to the point response, out of an overriding concern for maintaining harmony. . . . Achieving harmony between conflicting and seemingly contradictory beliefs follows from a long tradition. A large part of this belief system has its origins in Indonesian religious beliefs and cosmology. . . . The "state ideology" of Pancasila, . . . the belief in authoritarian and hierarchical structures, that people should know and stay in their place, the appropriateness of behaviors as tied to social status, and the fixed nature of one's destiny stands in opposition to such [self-]development. (1989:24–25)

Many Asian cultures promote passivity. The streets of India are filled with people—with and without disabilities—who are begging. The problem is not that people are begging but the social conditions that create the need for it. Religion, the church, and the passivity they foster are part and parcel of these social conditions.

Franz Harsana Sasraningrad: "We [in Indonesia] don't like conflict. Our religion leads us to want harmony above everything else."

Rajendra Vyas: "Our religion helps us cope with our caste, our place on earth."

The relationship between religion and disability must be analyzed on two levels. First, what kind of message do various religious doctrines convey about disability? That is, do they contribute to or help break down the myths and stereotypes about disability? Second, what is the social and political role of religion as an institution? That is, does the church foster or hinder the movement for social justice? Ultimately, though there are exceptions, religion, the most influential ideological influence on attitudes and ideas, fails on both counts.

LANGUAGE AND THE POWER OF DESCRIPTION

We must take language very seriously. The feeling I have is that language is always a reflection of attitude. With the advancement of the disability movement you see a change in language.

> Michael Masutha, director of socioeconomic rights, Lawyers for Human Rights, Johannesburg, South Africa

Language informs attitudes and beliefs because it is a medium of translation of expression and thought. When a word or an idea is expressed, an image is generated. As the Russian linguist V. N. Volosinov suggests, "experience is organized" ([1930] 1973:85). When a term is used over and over again, it establishes a meaning, an image, a reality. An etymology of words about disability helps to trace the culturally based sources for many backward ideas about disability.[7] As Linda Nicholson points out, language is a social product: "Thus, many terms in our language, such as 'production,' 'mothering' and 'sex' are ambiguous between possessing a strictly limited physical meaning and possessing a more culturally loaded meaning" (1993:55). Not only is language affected by society and culture, society and culture are affected, reciprocally, by language. The kinds of images that terms like "cripple," "invalid," "retard," "confined to a wheelchair," "blind as a bat," and "deaf and dumb" generate have an ideological and therefore social and cultural impact. The words used to describe disability are loaded with social connotations. Language is regarded by many as the "most social" of all "social facts" (Schmidt 1985:53).

The meaning of disability as infirmity/deformity has a long history. This history is testimony to the force of language and its power of description. *Invalid, chirema, pena, minasvalida, ai duan*—all signify less human, innately inferior. They provide an ideological mechanism that subtly but convincingly dehumanizes people.

Ranga Mupindu: "In Africa, in our culture, we do not even use the awful term 'cripple.' It's even worse. In Shona, the word is *chirema*, which means totally useless, a failure. So a person with a disability begins life as a chirema."

In Zimbabwe, Shona and Ndebele are the two most common spoken languages. In Ndebele, the common term for a person with a disability is *isigoga,* which connotes helplessness. It means the person cannot do anything alone and must wait for assistance. In Shona, the term for a blind person is *bofu,* connoting someone without freedom. In Ndebele, the term for the blind is *isiphofu,* connoting helplessness. In Shona, the word for deafness is *matsi;* in Ndebele, *isacuthe.* Both refer to one who needs help, although the pejorative connotation is not strong in Shona. The term *ongezwayo,* meaning stubborn, is also used in Ndebele. No doubt all languages provide similar examples. Bernhard Helander writes that all the words used by the Hubeer in southern Somalia to describe particular disabilities connote illness (Ingstad and Whyte 1995:77–87).

Description of disability is not limited only to words that have a negative impact on attitudes about disability. The power of description manifests itself also through proverbs, slang and idioms, folklore, and legends. Besides the specific terms, a number of Shona and Ndebele proverbs use disability as an idiom of culture. They are illustrative. In Shona, *chirema chinemazano chinotamba chakazendama kumadziro* translates as "a disabled person can be clever and dance if he is leaning against a wall." It means all people have abilities as long as they try and seek help. It is similar to "God helps those who help themselves." Another common adage is *seka urema wafe,* or "laugh at disability when you are dead." It means do not tempt fate. In Ndebele, *ubulima kabuhlaleli* translates as "disability does not wait for anybody." A somewhat similar saying has a more pejorative effect: *okwehlela inja lemuntwini kuyafika,* "what may happen to a dog may happen to you tomorrow." This means do not think the disabled are stupid or despise them because the same may happen to you (UNILO 1993).

For the last two decades people with disabilities have waged a political, policy, legal, academic, and philosophical struggle to make disability-related language neutral and more responsive to the changing political and cultural world. This is a difficult and protracted struggle, as Stuart Hall reminds us: "Think of how profound it has been in our world to say the word 'Black' in a new way. In order to say 'Black' in a new way, we have to fight off everything else that Black has meant . . . the entire metaphorical structure of Christian thought, for example" (1991:10). Fortunately, in some places, we can distinguish a gradual transition of terms describing disability—from "cripple" to "handicapped," "disabled" to "person with a disability." These are important symbolic steps forward.

The struggle to change language describing disability is particularly interesting in Spanish. The most common expression in Latin America is *minasvalidas,* which translates as "less valid." The term *discapitados* (less capable) is also very common. Pejorative terminology about disability abounds in Spanish, and in fact, there is not one politically correct term describing disability in the dictionary. We in the disability rights movement created our own term, *personas con deshabilidades,* or persons with disabilities. The word *deshabilidades* is not in the dictionary. When people point this out, believing that this means we cannot use the word, we proudly tell them we will not accept the language of the oppressors just because some book perpetuates the stereotypes and myths we are fighting to break down. The DRM has targeted language as an important issue for just this reason.

Maria Paula Teperino: "Lots of work needs to be done with language. People usually call us *aliejado,* which means cripple. I believe inaccessibility has a lot to do with this because people see us being carried into buildings and they think we are sick."

Narong Patibatsarakich: "In Thailand, it doesn't matter what disability people are referring to, they always say *ai,* which means 'to look down on.' They say *ai duan* to refer to amputees, *ai bod* for people who are blind, *ai bah* for the mentally ill, and so on."

Danilo Delfin: "Language of course is important. There is the history of using slang like 'cripple' or 'useless.' In Filipino the word is *lumpo* or *inutil.* We try to emphasize 'with disability'—*may kapansanan* in Filipino; *con pikan* in Thai; *chon pika* in Kampuchean."

Everywhere in the world the issue of language appears to be illustrative of the position people with disabilities find themselves in. In China, people with disabilities have been historically called *canfei,* which means "crippled and useless." More recently, since the founding of the China Disabled Persons Federation (CDPF), the more neutral *canji,* "disabled," has appeared. The experience is similar in Asia, Africa, and Latin America since disability-related organizations have come under the control of people with disabilities. Ultimately, the language used to describe people with disabilities will change because it is now being actively contested by those it describes.

A Socialization Formula on Disability

I remember well a friend telling me when I was a teenager never to accept someone's pity because pity is the pleasure of the mediocre person.

Paulo Saturnino Figueiredo, activist,
Belo Horizonte, Brazil

People with disabilities are significantly affected by the way in which culture(s) explain the cause of their disabilities (God's will, reincarnation, witchcraft); the images disability evokes (the sick/deformed body); and how they are described (cripple, invalid, retard). These interact to produce the ways in which society at large is socialized to think about disability. Socialization works on simple symbols, simple repetition. Over and over the myth as message is repeated: disability = sickness/deformation; sickness = helpless and deformation = abomination; helpless = protection and abomination = asexuality; asexuality = childlike; childlike = helpless/protection; helpless/protection = pity; pity = disability. The message can be simplified: disability = invalid; invalid = inferior; inferior = disability. The logic is circular, but it works.

CHAPTER 5

Consciousness and Alienation

Demonstrating a phenomenology of disability oppression requires consideration of how the relations and structures of that oppression are reproduced. In examining these relationships, many considerations unfold from the central questions of how people think about, feel, and cope with the particular manifestation of that oppression in their own lives and—more simply—why people passively consent to power. Are they manipulated or co-opted? Scared or apathetic? Can they not control their lives, or do they have no hope and vision of such control?

The short answer might be, various combinations of these. But we also know that wherever oppression has existed, there has been resistance to it. Both sides of this dynamic, passivity and resistance, are bound up with people's own consciousness about themselves and the world they live in.

As I discussed in chapter 2, there are two crucially interconnected aspects of this dynamic: hegemony, the embracing of the dominant belief system that naturalizes superiority and inferiority, power and powerlessness; and alienation, the internalization of oppression that creates an emasculation of the self. How hegemony and alienation operate both in societies and on individuals reveals a lot about why, how, and who acquiesces to and resists oppression.

Georg Lukács is widely recognized as the first to analyze the psychological impact of the integration of political economy and dominant culture. In one of his most often quoted passages, he argues that people's own ideas become transformed into an objectified worldview as a psychological by-product of the integration of the processes of capitalist production and culture:

The transformation of the commodity relation into a thing of ghostly objectivity cannot therefore content itself with the reduction of all objects for the gratification of human needs to commodities. It stamps its imprint upon the whole consciousness of people; their qualities and abilities are no longer an organic part of their personality, they are things which people can "own" or "dispose of" like the various objects of the external world. And there is no natural form in which human relations can be cast, no way in which people can bring their physical and psychic qualities into play without their being subjected increasingly to this reifying process. (1971:100)

Real individual needs and desires vanish, and only the "reified" ideas allowed by that objectified worldview exist. Individuals lose their humanity, and their "worth" becomes dependent on their profitability—Lukács's "ghostly objectivity." A process of reification unfolds as people become estranged from their own self and others as well. They experience a paralyzing alienation.

We can observe this process in people with disabilities. Their evolution of consciousness is informed for the most part by lives of economic and social deprivation in which they are told every day, in one way or another, that they are pathetic, grotesque, and, most significant, inferior. This message is reinforced by a variety of social institutions. Families hide them, tell them they will always be dependents. Those lucky enough to attend school are segregated and taught they are *special* (read: inferior). Religion attributes disability to atonement, reincarnation, sin, or the lack of ancestor worship. The media portrays people with disabilities as helpless and/or angry, maladjusted cripples. They are dehumanized and their worth is reduced to cost-benefit analyses and the balance sheets of the companies that provide "special" services to them.

Although the sociopolitical implications of this totality are profound (isolation, poverty, etc.), the psychological ramifications are just as significant. Society's backward beliefs about and attitudes toward disability not only are society's beliefs; they are internalized by most people with disabilities as well. This explains why consciousness, or more precisely, the *falsification* of it, is not only a crucial element in the oppression of people with disabilities but also the major barrier faced by the disability rights movement.

Power(lessness) and (False) Consciousness

Most consent to the existing power structure not just because they have embraced its values. People also internalize oppression to such an extent that they do not believe they are capable of such things as making production decisions, influencing political and social trends, and participating in policy making. Many, as Marx contends in *Capital,* are so beaten down that they see no hope of controlling their lives: "The class of the proletariat feels annihilated in its self-alienation; it sees its own powerlessness and the reality of an inhuman existence" ([1867] 1964a, 3:691). This is the case for people with disabilities. Theirs is an alienation that is both experienced and expressed in terms of self-pity and self-doubt as well as fear and shame. Although many individuals have broken free of this personal annihilation, most have not. I believe that the feeling of inferiority is the principal reason people with disabilities have not confronted and contested power and their own powerlessness. Alienation is both a consequence of the grinding degradation of oppression and exploitation and its indispensable handmaid, dehumanization (commodification), which hides or justifies its existence.

There is an old story that is illustrative of the relationship between labor and alienation. A coal miner's daughter asks her father why they do not have any coal left to keep the house warm. The father replies, "Because I have been laid off at work and we cannot afford coal." She pursues her questioning: "Why were you laid off at work, daddy?" He responds: "They said the price of coal has fallen so much they cannot make enough to keep us on." "But daddy, why did the price of coal drop? It's so necessary." The father now somewhat ashamedly says: "They say that too much coal was mined, and now there is glut of it, they can't sell it all." He turns away, but his daughter makes a remarkable conclusion: "You say we don't have any coal because the boss has too much!" "Yes, that's it, honey." "But why don't they just give us some if they have more than they can use?" "Because," says the father, "that's not the way things work."

This story illustrates what Bertell Ollman calls "alienated labor" or "the alienated character of use-value" (1971:185). In it we find three insights. First, the worker, having lost control of her labor and her work product, loses any chance to control her own needs, in this case a warm house. Second, this separation of actual work from work product (what the worker produces is not hers) hides the worker's commodification/dehumanization from herself. Third, it reveals the dual nature of commodities (use value/exchange value, in this case labor power and coal). Work always has use value, work is useful. But it does not always have an exchange value (people are unemployed because the market does not need or value what they can sell, their labor power). In this example, coal is always useful, but sometimes it cannot be exchanged, making its value useless. Herbert Marcuse, in paraphrasing Marx, puts it simply: "Workers become poorer the more wealth they produce" (1964:277).

Marx wrote extensively on alienation because he recognized its link to (false) consciousness and powerlessness. Like other social groups whose alienation is derived from the lack of control they have over their own lives, Marx locates the genesis of workers' alienation at the moment they lose control of their own labor power: "But the exercise of labor power, labor, is the worker's own life-activity, the manifestation of his own life. And this life-activity he sells to another person in order to secure the necessary means of subsistence. Thus his life-activity is for him only a means to enable him to exist. He works in order to live. He does not even reckon labor as part of his life, it is rather a sacrifice of his life" (Meszaros 1970:122).[1]

In the workplace we can see the relationship between hegemony and alienation. On the one hand, it is necessary to legitimate and naturalize the hierarchies of and separation between owner, manager, supervisor, and worker. On the other hand, work is one of the most highly social and collaborative activities in which people are engaged. Many labor scholars have shown how this separation (estrangement) and isolation process involves deskilling; greater differentiation of tasks; part-time workers; and less responsibilities and less autonomy (creativity) through increased supervision. In his groundbreaking and controversial book, *Labor and Monopoly Capitalism,* Harry Braverman argued that deskilling is part and parcel of workers' self-annihilation and acquiescence to the hegemonic position of the bosses.[2]

I have introduced Marx's concept of alienation for two reasons. First, he is most closely associated with the theory of alienation. Second, and more important, the key to understanding the implications of alienation in a world system dominated by capital is to recognize its dehumanizing and isolating qualities. Istvan Meszaros, in *Marx's Theory of Alienation*, emphasizes that the separation and isolation of the individual from the social body is the central feature of the process of alienation: "characterized by the universal extension of 'saleability'; by the conversion of human beings into 'things' so that they could appear as commodities on the market; and by the fragmentation of the social body into 'isolated individuals'" (1970:35).

Alienation unfolds over a long time. It involves the everyday experiences of individual people in their own homes and communities, at work, in schools; as women, as workers, as colonized peoples, and as people with disabilities. Alienation is similar to hegemony in its organic link to the institutions and realities of everyday life as well as its psychological outcome—hopelessness, rationalization of oppression, and the inconceivability of power. Hegemony's relationship to alienation can be simply summarized: hegemony relates to power *in the context of ideas* like alienation relates to ideas *in the context of power.*

(False) Consciousness, Alienation, and Disability Oppression

We, the disabled, have assimilated a consciousness in which we think we are unable to do this or that. That is, we deserve help, pity. All we do is request. And when you think only of requesting help, you put yourself in a position of begging. You are always begging, not only for money. People with disabilities have never sought for their own, although we have started doing it nowadays. You are the mirror of society. If you think of yourself as inferior, people will relate to you as if they are superior. If we do not overcome this individualist attitude we have, we will continue to be the target of charity. This can only be overcome through political activism. Otherwise we will be paralyzed.

> Arnaldo Godoy, Belo Horizonte [Brazil] City
> Council member

As a child, I noticed disparities between black and white. I knew whites were much better off. I was raised to believe whites were superior and blacks weren't achievers. I truly believed whites were superior. I never hated whites, I respected them for their natural superiority. . . . Whites were large farmers, blacks were subsistence farmers. I grew up in a rural area. I just believed it was correct. My school was run

by whites, and there I learned of white people's incompetence.
I was shocked to find that whites failed at things and didn't
know things. I think these same lessons can be applied to the
disabled. We are always taught we are inferior.

Michael Masutha, Disabled People South Africa

In *Black Skin, White Masks* Frantz Fanon examined the effects of colonization on the colonized. His influential work described
the "psychic alienation of the black man" (1967:12) and exposed the
colonialist mythology that dehumanized the "native" and "civilized" the
oppressor. He then argued that only until the colonized recognized this
self-alienation could they develop a consciousness of liberation. Reading Fanon from the perspective of disability oppression, the parallels are
irresistible. For instance, Fanon's discussion of the impact of language
on Algerians: "Every French expression referring to the Algerian had a
humiliating content. Every French speech heard was an order, a threat,
or an insult" (1965:89). Dehumanization is complicated. At times it is
subtle, at other times not so subtle. Consider two signs:

WHITES ONLY, COLORED USE OTHER ENTRANCE

ELEVATORS FOR FREIGHT AND HANDICAPPED ONLY—PLEASE USE STAIRS

When highlighted in the text of a book, the discrimination and degradation these signs promote are blatant. They dehumanize. More widespread in today's world is the coding of prejudice and discrimination.

Maria da Comceição Caussat: "Another example of disability discrimination is in the employment ads that say, 'Good Appearance Required.' In
Brazil, this is a code for no disabled and no blacks. I think these advertisements affect peoples' attitudes about themselves and also support society's
prejudice."

For another set of examples, I return to Fanon. Fanon's critique of
the psychological impact of colonial domination parallels the DRM's critique of disability mythology. The alienation from oneself and from others that Fanon situates in education, language, and sexuality is strikingly
familiar to the writings coming out of the DRM.

For Fanon, the conditions for emancipation start with the "struggle
against the mechanisms of concealment." The colonized are alienated
from each other through the ideology of racism that hides from them

and their humanity and potential as people and their interests and commonalities as oppressed people. In her book on Fanon, Renate Zahar explains, "The white society in which he lives constantly reminds the black man of his being different, either by friendly curiosity or overpoliteness or by outright discrimination. The white man's attitude toward blacks tends to show the features of adult behavior towards children. . . . Often this type of discrimination is unintentional and casual, but it is the very matter-of-factness and indifference of such behavior which most emphatically shows the Negro his place" (1974:29).

Just change Zahar's quote slightly: The majority of society constantly reminds us we are different, either by friendly curiosity (pats on the head, staring, pointing) or overpoliteness ("let me do that for you") or outright discrimination ("we don't rent to people like you"). Society's attitudes toward people with disabilities tend to show the features of adult behavior toward children (the waiter asking a companion, "What does he want to eat?" or the airline steward, "How does she want me to help her?"). Often this type of discrimination is unintentional and casual, but it is the very matter-of-factness and indifference of such behavior that most emphatically shows the person with a disability his or her place.

Moreover, as the process of dehumanization unfolds over time, it informs, even conditions, behaviors that oppressed people encounter in others. This may include insults and ridicule, physical attacks, stares, avoidance, and being patronized. In *Femininity and Domination*, Sandra Bartky postulates a phenomenology of women's oppression. In one passage she describes a familiar scenario: "It is a fine spring day, and with an utter lack of self-consciousness, I am bouncing down the street. Suddenly I hear men's voices. Catcalls and whistles fill the air. These noises are clearly sexual in intent and they are meant for me; they come from across the street. I freeze. . . . The body which only a moment before I inhabited with such ease now floods my consciousness. I have been made into an object" (1990:21). This passage illuminates the link between dehumanization and objectification.

A phenomenology of oppression and self-alienation exists for people with disabilities. Our community's history of isolation, degradation, dependency, medicalization, and discrimination has created an internalized alienation of self-pity and inferiority akin to other oppressed groups. People with disabilities are objectified and conditioned in ways that are similar to the experience of other oppressed groups.

In *No More Stares,* women with disabilities chronicle objectification:

If I had one wish, it would be that people realized how their staring hurts me, and that I can't help being small. I was just made that way. I guess others just don't know how it makes me feel . . . or else why would they stare? (Ginny)

When I was younger, I was extremely aware that someone was staring at me, even though I couldn't see. If I made a mistake and ran into a tree, someone would see me. Someone would know that I wasn't "normal." (Sheila) (Carrillo, Corbett, and Lewis 1982:11)

Oppression negates one's humanity. Again, from *No More Stares:*

Sometimes I feel really alone because of my disability. I am hard of hearing and although I can function fairly well in both the hearing and the deaf worlds, I do not, at times, feel a part of either world. I am not totally accepted as deaf because I can talk and lip-read fairly well, and I am not totally accepted as hearing because there are times when I cannot hear and use an interpreter. (Missy)

Early in my disability I had a rejecting attitude towards other disabled and have only just got rid of this. I didn't want to mix with disabled people, didn't want to be associated with them. I wanted to pass for non-disabled. . . . I wanted desperately to be accepted as "normal." (Elsa) (Ibid., 15)

The self-pity and insularity people with disabilities experience are not simply a phenomenon of underdevelopment. These are North American women. People with disabilities have a history of isolation and self-pity that transcends center/periphery boundaries. These experiences, though, are very common as minority experiences, as experiences of oppression.

Juxtapose *No More Stares* to Renate Zahar's summary of Fanon's theory of alienation: "The colonized man is *handicapped* (my emphasis; her term) in establishing contacts with his environment through his complexes and feelings of insecurity; by and by he becomes, in Fanon's phrase, the 'prisoner of an unbearable insularity.' Any possible way out of this solitude inevitably leads him into the white world" (1974:51). Dehumanization produces different outcomes. Most immediately one feels an alienation from self and others resulting in self-pity, low esteem, and insecurity. Fanon captures this well: "I slip into corners, I remain silent, I strive for anonymity, for invisibility. Look, I will accept my lot, as long as no one notices me!" (Fanon 1967:116). Fanon's characterization mirrors the next passage from *No More Stares*:

People stare at you if you're different. They can make you feel like a Martian. I never really wanted to go out because I was so self-conscious. My family would say, "You have to go out, we'll take you to the beach." I wouldn't. So my father would get off work at night and we'd go to the movies. The only show I'd go to was the late show that started at 10:00 o'clock. It was dark in the streets and in the theater. My father would wheel me out as soon as the lights came up. (Carrillo, Corbett, and Lewis 1982:11)

Two related consequences of alienation are the obscuration of oppression and the elimination of real identity. Oppressed people tend to blame themselves for conditions over which they have little control. They feel helpless and hopeless, which often produces a tragic nihilism of misdirected hate and anger. Cornel West describes the nihilism fostered in African-American communities in the United States as "the lived experience of coping with a life of horrifying meaninglessness, hopelessness, and [most important] lovelessness" (1993:14).

Nihilism is an important aspect of oppression. It is a form of alienation in its most desperate stage. Its social manifestations—suicide, crime, domestic violence, alcoholism, drug abuse—conceal one's oppression from one's own self. Meaninglessness, hopelessness, and lovelessness are often felt by people with disabilities. Alienation and false consciousness reflect real-life conditions. People do not feel meaningless, hopeless, and loveless because they are detached from reality, but because the realities of their everyday life provide them with little reason to be hopeful or feel their life has meaning, and they may, in fact, be unloved. This nihilism, as West defines it, is a reasonable response to poverty and powerlessness, isolation and degradation.

Alienation also makes it difficult to identify with other people in similar circumstances. Estranged individuals do not want to be who they are. They, as Sartre said, take themselves for somebody else. This self-deception is insidious. Fanon saw this lack of recognition or lack of identification as a fundamental ideological barrier to liberation. In perhaps the most famous passage in *Black Skin, White Masks*, Fanon unmasks this failure of recognition: "Attend a showing of a Tarzan film in the Antilles and in Europe. In the Antilles, the young Negro identifies himself de facto with Tarzan against the Negroes. This is much more difficult for him in a European theater, for the rest of the audience, which is white, automatically identifies him with the savages on the screen" (1967:152–153).

Power and Ideology: The Implications of (False) Consciousness for Identity (and Its Failure)

In searching for answers to the elusive questions concerning consciousness formation, many contemporary political writers have asserted the centrality of identification. As Ernesto Laclau writes, "When Lacoue-Labarthe asks, 'Why, after all, should the problem of identification not be, in general, the essential problem of politics?' we could add that the problem is not identification, but identification and *its failure*" (1994:35). This ranges from how and why women or religious or racial groups relate to each other (or do not) to the development of nationalism. Each of these and the myriad other ways in which people identify themselves (as an auto worker, musician, mother, stamp collector, sports fan, etc.) have their own particular defining qualities.

Questions about identity and the lack of identity are complex and powerful: Why do people, based on particular identities, hate and even kill people of different identities? Why do some groups more easily identify with each other? Are all identities contrived? Is identity formation primarily economic, psychological, cultural, or political? If identity formation is not the central issue of politics, then certainly it is among the most important.

Just as certain is the dilemma posed by the failure of disability identification for the disability rights movement: "People with disabilities have, for the most part, failed to identify with each other as a group. This has been detrimental because it has built a sense of isolation when a camaraderie based upon existing commonalities could have been developed" (Brown 1992:227). The failure of most people with disabilities to identify with other people with disabilities is, I believe, the principal contradiction that limits the DRM's potential influence and power.

It should not be surprising that oppressed people do not typically relate to and identify with their oppression, either as individuals or in a group. All the signposts of their lives point them away from this kind of consciousness. Part and parcel of oppression is the shame of inferiority. This is especially true in a world that is individualistic and fragmented, bombastic and image conscious. Furthermore, for the overwhelming majority of people the simple struggle to survive is exhausting. It is hard to see beyond the necessities and vulgarities of each day.

To analyze why people with disabilities have not identified with disability, it may be useful to contrast other oppressed groups that have strong bonds of self-identification. For example, the Palestinians are among the most oppressed and fragmented groups, yet their group identity is extremely cohesive. Whether they live in the West Bank, in London, or in Detroit, Palestinians proudly identify themselves as Palestinian.[3] In his article, "A Country of Words: Conceiving the Palestinian Nation from the Position of Exile," Glenn Bowman argues that Palestinian identification is bound together by stories, songs, and, most important, imagination: "It is a central contention . . . that all ideas of community are 'imaginary' constructions in so far as community always exists through the imaging of the group of which one conceives oneself a member. Darwish's phrase, 'a country of words,' has pertinence not only to Palestinians and others who have suffered from nation theft and can only locate their countries in reminiscences, stories, songs and histories, but also to those who, living within existent communities, take the presence of those entities as given" (1994:140). Bowman's emphasis is on discursive politics, the formation of political identities through histories, through words and communication—what he calls the "obsessive re-creation of the past" (ibid., 148). He goes on to show the inherent limitations to identities forged without common experiences and based in discourse. He quotes from Edward Said's *After the Last Sky* to make his point: "Intimate mementoes of a past irrevocably lost circulate among us, like the genealogies and fables severed from the original locale, the rituals of speech and custom. Much reproduced, enlarged, thematized, embroidered and passed around, they are strands in the web of affiliations we Palestinians use to tie ourselves to our identity and to each other" (ibid., 151).

Much that Bowman says applies to disability identification and its failure. First, self-identification with disability is difficult because there is no history of disability—it has not been written and it is not known—nor is it acknowledged. Second, one cannot "imagine" something that does not exist—a disabled community. Our community is isolated, scattered, and without a positive signification (who would want to self-identify as a cripple, an invalid?). Third, there has never been a disability culture passed down in families or by other means through stories, customs, and language.[4] Fourth, people with disabilities have not had a "web of affiliations" to relate to and get support from. Finally, it needs to be emphasized that as an amalgam of similar and divergent characteristics, people with disabilities potentially have multiple, partially overlapping, and semicontradictory identities. We could and sometimes do take on an identity based on a combination of factors such as our own specific disability; our homeland or ethnicity (as Mexicans or Latin Americans, Zimbabweans or Africans, Chinese or Asians); or even the disability organization or issue we relate to. Identity formation is further (and often primarily) influenced by class, race, gender, or sexual orientation. It is in each of these areas—historiography, culture, signification, affiliation, and difference—that identification and its failure are revealed.

The Implications of (False) Consciousness for the Disability Rights Movement

Powerlessness and false consciousness reinforce each other; the failure of disability identification reinforces both. The implications are decisive for the disability rights movement. For without raised consciousness on the part of people with disabilities, there will not be a powerful disability rights movement, and without a powerful DRM, there will not be mass consciousness about disability. The DRM has, from the beginning, recognized this contradiction and tried to address itself to the implications of disability identification and its failure. Only recently, however, have activists thoroughly considered the complexity of this problem.

First, disability rights activists have begun to establish histories of disability. This effort has ranged from articles and books on individual lives to broader histories. Each of these addresses disability from the perspective of people who have lived it. Newsletters and journals are being circulated. From these efforts, a common heritage of disability has begun to be constructed.[5]

Second, a disability culture is emerging. Music is being written, performed, recorded, and distributed. Troupes of dancers with disabilities have toured, and stage plays have been produced. There is a growing body of literature as well. Athletics has become the most popular expression of this phenomenon, encompassing all sports events.

Third, there has been a serious and partially successful effort to change the way people with disabilities are referred to. The DRM has correctly recognized the power of description as a way to unlock some of the doors that block self-identification. As Steven Brown, a disability rights activist who has paid a great deal of attention to issues of disability identification and culture, writes, "During the past ten to twenty years, there has been a great deal of discussion about appropriate language to use when discussing disability. . . . [A]ll groups search for definitions of identity. The debate about what we call ourselves, the discussion surrounding language, represents a corner piece in the jigsaw puzzle of our beliefs about ourselves and who we are" (1992:5). There is an international effort to change the discourse of disability. Identity has to be positively imagined before it will be fully formed.

Fourth, thousands of disability-related organizations, support groups, and self-help projects have materialized in less than two decades which can serve as webs of affiliation for people with disabilities. These range from an individual person coordinating a support group to large nongovernmental organizations with a significant budget and staff. There are also important international confederations and policy and development groups.

Fifth, the disability rights movement has recognized both the commonalities and differences among people with disabilities. The DRM has recognized that to be successful in positively mediating the gap between false consciousness and a collective identity, it must be able to reach out to different people in different circumstances and stimulate them to reach out to others.

The key to unlocking the dilemma of identification and its failure lies in the phenomenology of oppression itself. Fundamentally, identities are contrived because they only exist as products of domination. Social groups exist as collectors of people whom the dominant culture selects for exclusion. Manning Marable elaborates by articulating the relation of race to class:

Ironically, the historical meaning and reality of race was always fundamentally a product of class domination. Race, in the last analysis, is neither biologically nor genetically derived. It is a structure rooted in white supremacy, economic exploitation, and social privilege. It evolved in the process of slavery and the transatlantic slave trade. Racism has power only as a set of institutional arrangements and social outcomes which perpetuate the exploitation of black labor, and the subordination of the black community's social and cultural life. (1995:72)

Race has little to do with skin color differences and everything to do with being oppressed for political-economic and sociocultural reasons.

Racism is not a set of backward attitudes about people of other skin colors, it is the product of a dominant culture, a domination that logically exploits, oppresses, and degrades people.

This point holds true for people with disabilities as well. The oppression of people with disabilities does not derive from a backward set of attitudes about disability, it is the product of a dominant culture that marginalizes people in the process of domination. Disability identification takes place as people begin to recognize their oppression. Oppression structures consciousness. It imbues consciousness with experiences of oppression. Whether a person relates to and identifies himself or herself with his or her oppression as a person with a disability, an African-American, a woman, a man, a worker, a Palestinian, a South African, or a mixture of these, flows out of the individual experience with oppression. Only when the DRM organizes around these experiences of oppression can they affect the consciousness and identification of members in its community. This has little to do with defining who is disabled. It has to do with people recognizing their common experiences as oppressed people. This is crucial for the development of raised consciousness, which in turn is necessary for empowerment. Ultimately, the DRM must recognize that the phenomenology of oppression is a totality of lived experiences—from poverty and isolation to cultural degradation and self-pity. The oppression that produces powerlessness and false consciousness is systemic and not simply the representation of outdated attitudes of those who do not know any better. The experiences of oppression are not only particular to the site of oppression (the asylum, the charity, the classroom), they are generalized throughout society by the necessity to reproduce the existing power relations. In effect, oppression has a logic that creates formidable barriers to raised consciousness through its economic, social, and cultural formations and institutions and at the same time creates the necessity and impulse for political activism. It is oppression itself that has created the everyday lived experiences out of which disability rights activists have emerged. Oppression has always engendered both passivity and resistance.

CHAPTER 6

Observations on Everyday Life

The first volume of Fernand Braudel's magnum opus, *Civilization and Capitalism, 15th–18th Century,* examines everyday life because everyday life is the context, medium, and range of what was possible for people during these centuries. In this book, Braudel studies subjects as diverse as what people ate and wore to the kinds of economic exchange they used. Although Braudel recognized the insights that resulted for what they were—"snapshots" of or portholes into the lives of real people—he nevertheless upheld their validity: "Everyday life consists of the little things one hardly notices in time and space. . . . Through the travellers' notes, a society stands revealed. The ways people eat, dress, or lodge, at the different levels of that society, are never a matter of indifference. And these snapshots can also point out contrasts and disparities between one society and another which are not at all superficial. It is fascinating, and I do not think pointless to try and reassemble these imageries" (1979:29). This is what I have set out to do here as well, recognizing, as Braudel does, the inherent limitations of such observations.

As I have suggested in preceding chapters, the overarching structures of everyday life for people with disabilities are poverty, powerlessness, and backward attitudes (degradation). These structures erect what Braudel called the "limits of the possible" for the vast majority of people with disabilities. But it is necessary to provide more than simply this general conceptual perspective of disability oppression, because all oppressed peoples experience these conditions.

In this chapter I describe seven additional features of everyday life that provide a more vivid and complete representation of the limits of the possible for people with disabilities: (1) invisibility; (2) lack of support services; (3) control by charities; (4) hierarchy of disability; (5) vulnerability to violence; (6) inaccessibility; and (7) chasm between rural and urban life. These features have their own peculiar relationships with poverty, powerlessness, and backward attitudes and with each other.

Invisibility and Abandonment

A few years ago we found out that the director-general of public welfare, who is responsible for rehabilitation [in Thailand], had a daughter who was mentally retarded. She had not received any rehabilitation services. She was hidden at home because he was ashamed of her.

Narong Patibatsarakich, chairperson, Disabled Peoples' International Thailand

People with disabilities are invisible and anonymous. Their situation brings to mind Ralph Ellison's famous passage in *Invisible Man*: "I am an invisible man. No, I am not a spook. . . . I am a man of substance, of flesh and bone, fiber and liquids—and I might even be said to possess a mind. I am invisible, understand, simply because people refuse to see me" ([1947]1989:3). There are three major reasons for this phenomenon: people with disabilities are often abandoned, hidden, and shunned by their own families and communities; segregation and inaccessibility have prevented people with disabilities from conducting fully public lives; extraordinary sociocultural stigmas have been brought to bear on those who have disabilities that are not readily apparent, so that they tend to conceal these disabilities from others. This is the case throughout the world, although the consequences are experienced differently depending on political-economic and sociocultural circumstances.

In the periphery, disability rights activists intuitively make the connections between isolation, endemic backward attitudes, and the hallmarks of underdevelopment—violence, poverty, and colonialism.

Paulo Saturnino Figueiredo: "The number of disabled people has never decreased in Brazil despite the control of poliomyelitis. The problem is much deeper. It is structural. It is a question of economics. I don't know if society unconsciously needs a mass of people with disabilities, but the lack of prevention is a scandal. This is the case especially in civil construction, where accidents are very common and responsible for the highest number of paraplegics due to construction companies' concern only for profits and not the safety of workers. Those people then disappear. When they don't die, they are taken to small cities or are put in the back part of a hut in a shantytown until they get rotten and die."

Koesbiono Sarmanhadi: "Children with disabilities are hidden because of an inferiority complex of families. This is attributable to a lack of education, which in turn is connected to Indonesia's level of poverty, our poor development. This is particularly the case in rural areas. The roots of this problem go back to the Dutch. Indonesia was colonized by the Dutch for three centuries, and they did nothing to improve the lives of the people, they only took."

Danilo Delfin: "I interviewed a Khmer Rouge soldier in Phenom Penh who said a big problem for disabled soldiers is that their wives abandon them because they don't want their families in the villages to find out their husbands are disabled."

Fernando Rodriguez: "By and large, people with disabilities in Mexico are very isolated, both because of their family's attitudes and because of all the access issues. Of course, people with disabilities who have money do not experience these problems in the same way because they can pay for transportation, for help to get into buildings, and so on. In my country, independent living really does not exist. The primary reasons for this are backward attitudes and the lack of economic development."

Over the years I have randomly surveyed people in various settings and circumstances. One question I always ask is, "Do you notice more blind people or people using wheelchairs about these days than ten years ago?" The typical answer is, "Yes. I never used to see these people by themselves." But if I press the point further, for example, "When was the last time you saw a person with a disability?" or "What are their names, and how can I get in touch with them?" the answer is, "I don't know." These responses show two things are occurring with regard to the issue of the (in)visibility of people with disabilities. First, the perception that more people are out and about is true; but, second, while the percentage increase of "visible" people with disabilities may be very large, the absolute number of people with disabilities going to school, shopping, getting married, going to parties, playing sports, and going for walks is still quite small.

Jerome Mindes's study of international efforts to improve rehabilitation services in China indicates that a formidable obstacle to such improvement is precisely the isolation of people who are in need of these services: "In China, it is not uncommon to hear of mentally ill or retarded adults who have lived their entire lives in back rooms, isolated from all but their immediate family. In rural areas, and even in the city of Beijing, one still hears anecdotal reference to children who are discarded at birth, and allowed to die of starvation" (1991:5).

Frequently, families are desperately hungry and cannot afford dependents. A graduate student at Beijing University summed this up for a Western journalist: "We want children to maintain the family line and support their parents in their old age. Disabled children are useless for either purpose so they become a luxury. Few people can afford luxuries in China" (*Chicago Tribune,* January 17, 1995). Asia is not alone.

Alexander Phiri: "After my accident, my parents visited two or three times and then I was abandoned. When I was to leave the hospital, the hospital people tried to locate my parents but failed. It was clear that they did not want a child they considered useless. Families have lots of children in Africa to increase the chances that one of their children will get a good job and provide for them when they are old. My parents thought I would only be a burden. They also did not want to deal with the social implications in their village for having a disabled child, because they would be ostracized and maybe even ridiculed."

Friday Mandla Mavuso: "In fact, [in Soweto, South Africa] a lot of people just gave up and wanted to stay in the hospital. . . . People even purposely developed bed sores to stay in the hospital. . . . Older paraplegics, for example, would tell new disabled that outside was suicide."

Abandonment is a huge social problem generally but especially affects children with disabilities. Out of a population of 143 million, Brazil has an estimated 20 million to 30 million abandoned children, some living in institutions but most wandering the streets of Rio, São Paulo, Recife, Salvador, and Belo Horizonte. An inordinate number of these children have disabilities. Life is so precarious in the Third World that a woman who has a baby with a disability is often deserted.

Rosangela Berman Bieler: "Vera Henriques, married for twenty years and mother of a fourteen-year-old girl with cerebral palsy, told me that she believes the vast majority of women with disabled children are abandoned by their husbands or companions because they do not accept the child's disability and they are so poor."

There is such poverty in the world that millions of people with disabilities are simply lost to society. They are invisible people. Narong Patibatsarakich's comments at the beginning of this section illustrate the centrality of isolation and invisibility in the everyday lives of people. If a person with a disability from a politically connected family cannot get the resources (which are extremely limited) they need to develop their potentialities because of backward attitudes, how will the hundreds of millions of poor, powerless people with disabilities get them? They will not, and they do not.

Surviving without a Safety Net

The structure of Brazilian society is reproduced within the disability community. Of the many lessons that disabled Brazilians could teach citizens from other countries, perhaps the most striking is how to survive in a society where there is no social safety net.

Eugene Williams, "Surviving Without a Safety Net in Brazil"

Appropriate support systems and technology such as brailling equipment and computers, wheelchairs and prosthetics, sign-language interpreters, and rehabilitation and psychiatric services exist but are available only to a small percentage of people with disabilities. This is primarily the case for Third World countries, although there is a wide disparity of support systems in the economically advanced regions. For example, northern Europe's safety net is far superior to anything in the United States, the rest of Europe, or Japan. In the United States there are significant differences between states and even within states.[1] With hundreds of millions of people with disabilities worldwide, a large demand exists for these services and supports.

People who need mobility aids, such as wheelchairs, braces, walkers, or prosthetics, often cannot secure appropriate sizes and many times cannot acquire any at all. This is an especially acute problem in Kampuchea, Afghanistan, Angola, and Egypt where there are millions of land mines and hundreds of thousands of people without limbs.[2] Wheelchairs, while available in most places, are almost always outmoded and unreliable. This is not simply a modest hindrance. It is a blatant violation of what should be a basic human right. Thanks to the efforts of activists like Ralf

Hotchkiss, who has promoted the design and construction of wheel-chairs internationally with locally available materials, there have been advances in the devices available to people with disabilities. As recently as the 1980s, common mobility aids were skateboardlike devices that people sat on and pushed along with their hands. The advantages of these were twofold: they were cheap (homemade), and they could traverse environmental and architectural barriers like steps and curbs. However, they are dangerous especially in the streets because drivers often cannot see people low to the ground; they are extremely dirty; the user must remain in a sitting position, which is very bad for the body; they are very slow; and they obscure the user's vision, making the disabled person more susceptible to attack. Most obvious is that they are thoroughly degrading. These devices, although not common, are still used today.

A device seen in Africa is the wheelchair-like tricycle. These rolling carts are relatively inexpensive as they are built with locally available materials. They are operated by peddling the chair with the hands. They can traverse rough terrain better than can traditional wheelchairs. In Kenya, I met Kenneth Moi, who essentially lived on the street in his tricycle. He told me his life is precarious and fragile because every time a tire or axle breaks he has to locate someone who will voluntarily repair his tricycle or give him simple parts, which he cannot afford.

Those with sensory and other hidden disabilities find a dearth of communication supports and aids. This is the case even for those with some financial resources. Brailling equipment, sign-language interpreters, and telecommunications technology like teletype telephones (TTYs) for the deaf do not even exist in many parts of the Third World. And there is no organized mobility training.

Charles Leung: "The blind throughout Asia, from what I have heard, do not have access to mobility training unless it is provided by family or friends."

Paradoxically, the area of everyday life that is both dissimilar and similar from one economic zone to another is education. In the periphery, education is simply unavailable to many children with disabilities. In contrast, in economically developed regions students with disabilities have access to some education, albeit a mostly degraded one. Here in the developed world, the educational experience of students labeled with the "special" status of "learning" disabled is particularly noteworthy, for they represent the greatest number of students with disabilities.

Nancy Ward: "When I was growing up in the fifties and sixties it was a very hard time for me. I was the oldest child in the family but all my brothers and sisters taught me how to do things like tie my shoes, eat, and get to school. I was in a regular classroom through the sixth grade. People would make fun of me, call me stupid, dummy, retard, and things, but I liked being in the regular classroom. The last day of sixth grade, the principal told me I was going into Special Ed. My parents knew this in advance but wouldn't even tell me. Education was just one labeling experience after another. I remember the grading system in high school. It was one to seven. Three was considered average, but the best people in Special Ed. could get was four. So, automatically we were considered less. We weren't even allowed to take history. In fact, when I was in high school I had to study from the same fifth-grade social studies textbook that I had in the regular classroom six years earlier. . . . My counselor was also head of Special Education. I remember doing a report in her office one day when another person walked in and they started talking about 'those mentally retarded people.' It was like I was not even there. I talked to the principal of the school about this but he said I was just overreacting. So these are some of the stories of my youth. . . . When I was to graduate I took a pre-nursing test at a local community college. On this test there were questions about algebra and calculus. It wasn't that I didn't know the answers to the algebra and calculus questions that bothered me. It was that I didn't even know what algebra and calculus were."

Indeed, the typical educational experience for young people with disabilities throughout the world is either outright exclusion or segregation. There are exceptions, of course, but segregating students from regular classrooms is common.

Hearing-impaired children face formidable barriers to obtaining a decent education. They are often mistakenly categorized as mentally retarded in early youth, which limits their intellectual and social development. Those who are "fortunate" are sent to segregated schools. In Third World countries, this usually means learning school-specific language codes and signs. For example, in South Africa, which has a very high standard of living for whites, there are only a handful of sign-language interpreters in the whole country. In addition, there are eight different sign-language systems in the country that developed at each of South Africa's deaf schools (until recently they were additionally segregated by race). This means a deaf adult in one region has a very difficult time communicating with a deaf person from another region. The impact of class is easily seen in the way this breaks down from one culture to another. The following is part of an interview with Susan Berde of the National Council of the Deaf in South Africa. Berde, who is white, comes from an affluent family.

Berde: "Later I moved to a deaf school in Rosebank, but signing was not allowed in school."

Q.: Signing was not allowed?

Berde: "No, not twenty years back. I was not able to improve my education because of this. . . . Then I went to Europe and to America for three years. I went to Gallaudet College in Washington. After three years I came back to South Africa because I did not have any more money for Gallaudet College. In South Africa, we have only a few TTYs but no captioning [on TV], no colleges, only a few interpreters, almost nothing for the deaf. It's very frustrating for me because I have been over there and have seen everything, and when I came back, it was terrible."

Q.: Over the years have you seen any changes?

Berde: "Some. Now, at school they're starting to have sign training for parents."

Q.: Well, how much access to interpreters is there for people who are deaf?

Berde: "There might be four or five, I think. Not enough for this country. They come from deaf families. There is no training. Last year we had a lecturer from the U.K. come to Durban University. She trained eighty people to teach hearing people sign language. We had an interpreter's workshop, but it was only one day in Durban."

Q.: What about black people who live in the countryside or who live in townships?

Berde: "There are quite a few African sign dialects I can understand. There are twelve dialects. Some signs are a little bit similar. But I cannot even tell which tribe, like Zulu or Tsosa, people come from. The issues for white and black deaf people are totally different. Our [whites'] biggest issue is getting TV subtitles. For black people, it's other things. One of their issues is to get a registration card with the Council because they get free bus service with it. White people don't really use it for that purpose. We have cars."

Q.: Are there any telephone relay services?

Berde: "No. We use Lifeline, which is a crisis hotline. There are many informal networks among us. This is the only way to find out things. We also have social clubs and get together every month. For people outside the bigger cities, there is nothing, I think."

The lack of support has significant social consequences for the deaf. It is common for the family to assign an older child responsibility to become an interpreter for a deaf sibling. If the person with the hearing disability is a parent, a child will be "trained" as an interpreter. This is not a sophisticated language but functional for everyday questions, responses, and needs. The results are problematic. The sibling or child interpreter becomes an appendage of the deaf sibling or parent. This often causes resentment in the family. The interpreter child resents being an "aid" instead of a brother or a daughter, and the parent feels indignant about his or her dependence on the child. It is, however, a necessity based on the limits of the possible.

There is an interesting and positive by-product of the segregation of deaf individuals, as Berde briefly mentions. As sign-language interpreters do not exist for all practical purposes and educational possibilities are limited, out of necessity deaf people often have a great deal of interaction with their deaf peers. Intricate communication networks that often amount to gossip, rumors, and interpersonal stories are widespread, although these are insular to the deaf community. It nevertheless is crucial to the ways in which deaf people survive. This is especially true of city dwellers. I would go so far as to say that deaf people, paradoxically, because of their cultural insularity, experience the most mobility and the broadest passing interaction with society and simultaneously the least real integration. When they enter the outside world, they do it in isolation because they have no means of communication access with that world. Here is an intersection where the isolated individual becomes invisible. Their world is silent. In a world without support, it is impenetrably silent.

Personal assistance is the crucial support that can often mean the difference between independence and dependence for people with significant physical disabilities. Personal assistants (PAs) might help people with getting out of bed in the morning, personal hygiene, cooking or shopping, and cleaning up. PAs often do tasks that would take a person with a disability a long time to do, thereby wasting both time and energy. These services, available to most people in economically developed regions, do not exist in the Third World. Furthermore, centers for independent living (CILs)—the principal promoters and deliverers of PA services in the United States—are very rare. The first such programs began in South America as recently as the early 1990s.

Rosangela Berman Bieler: "Before we started our center for independent living, personal assistance services did not exist in Brazil."

There are almost as many examples of life without the appropriate and necessary support as there are people with disabilities. Most activists conclude that of all people with disabilities, those with mental illness have the most difficult lives. This is the case throughout the world. We know that, with rare exceptions, the asylums of Europe and the United States are horrendous institutions. We also know that a sizable number of the homeless population in the United States have mental disabilities. Now for the bad news. For that, it is necessary to examine the range of options in the Third World. Setting aside questions about the value and role of professional mental health therapy, which I believe are dubious at best, it is illuminating to make such comparisons.

India, with its extraordinary population and poverty (alongside a relatively well developed professional strata), and the countries of Southeast Asia, with their booming economies, represent the two ends of the spectrum in Asia. With a national population now estimated at more than 900 million, India has only forty-two psychiatric hospitals with a combined capacity of 20,000 persons and a combined total of 2,500 mental health professionals (Dunlap 1990:70). The ASEAN region—Brunei, Indonesia, Malaysia, the Philippines, Thailand, and Singapore—has 650 psychiatrists for a population of 275 million, or approximately one psychiatrist for every half-million people (Deva 1990:22). The comparison shows that while the differences in level of service options for people with mental illness are unimpressive, the universal lack of resources is.

Charities and Social Services

Charities play a negative social role. They seek to control us. Charities are not interested in empowerment and integration. They support segregation. In fact, once we have integration and equalization of opportunity, these charities will begin to die. Their institutional interests lie with segregation, ours with integration.

Joshua Malinga, DPI/DPSA

My sister and I were Muscular Dystrophy Association poster children. Here we were back in 1962 and just kids and we were already being exploited by the Jerry Lewis telethon to pander to peoples' pity to raise money for their social services agency.

Mike Ervin, Chicago ADAPT

*In fact, when I moved to Sweden everyone just assumed I
moved here for the benefits and to go on welfare. The welfare
state with all its advantages to poor people has had a negative
effect on our movement to demand rights instead of services,
integration instead of segregation.*

Adolph Ratzka, director, Institute on Independent
Living, Stockholm

In Chapter 2 I suggested a way of thinking about how
(disability) oppression is rationalized and reproduced by focusing on the
role of ideology and ideological institutions in manufacturing consent
and, in the end, maintaining power and control. While the institutional
roles of schools, churches, and the media are relatively easy to recognize, there is one other, less obvious institution that functions as an
agency of control.

In what must be considered poignantly illustrative of their perilous
and degraded status, people with disabilities are significantly controlled
by charity and social service institutions (broadly considered, private welfare agencies, asylums, and residential facilities). This is the case throughout the world, although charities are more prevalent in the United States
and Europe. Rachel Hurst, a DPI leader from Great Britain, argues this
kind of control is colonialist in content: "There are organizations for
people with disabilities all over Europe but they are often subsumed under government or various charities' control. They are professional organizations, parent organizations, for example. They are barriers to giv-
ing our own voice to our issues. They cannot be radical. But the greatest
barrier of all is the charity ethic. Just as in Britain, all 'colonial' countries
are bristling with organizations run by professionals of one sort or another. The concept of consultation with disabled people has not been
on anyone's agenda—any more than consulting the natives was on their
agenda in their colonial past" (1995:530).

Many people argue that charity plays a positive role in the lives of the
"disadvantaged." Some might see that it is contradictory to point out
that most people with disabilities do not have access to a safety net while
at the same time criticizing charities and social service agencies. It is undoubtedly true that some individuals are helped by charities. But it is
precisely in this way that charities function as an agency of control. Charities, at best, create dependency; at worst, they further degrade and iso-
late. The raison d'être of charity is to help the helpless. Charities would
wither away, as Joshua Malinga points out, if people were not deemed
helpless by those who make such a determination. Charity is poverty's

silent subject. As dependency is a condition of oppression, charity is a condition of poverty.

Those who question the role of charities are considered maladjusted and too angry to know what is good for them. It is as if the oppressor would say, "You are impoverished and degraded so we have created this charity to take care of you. You should be grateful." This is reminiscent of Bertolt Brecht's famous line in *The Three Penny Opera*: "We would be good instead of being so rude, if only the circumstances were not of this kind." Billy Golfus in his article "The Do-gooder" echoes Malinga:

When I say Do-gooder, I don't just mean the counselors, staff, vocational personnel, and assorted "helpers." I mean the agencies, programs, or what they call "care providers." The term Do-gooders appears to suggest the kind of neighbor that brings over chicken soup when you're sick—and once in a while somebody'll even do that. But that's not what I mean. I guess, for the most part, I'm talking about the professionals. . . . After my accident, I started to have my eyes opened very slowly. It took me years, like they say, to process what had happened. While the physical disabilities and the brain damage that I have are inconvenient, a drag even, they're not as bad as the treatment by my friends, social systems and especially the Do-gooders. These people are "professionals," for God's sake. . . . To hang the word "helping" on "professional" gives the connotation of humanity, generosity, and compassion. As if their reasons for acting came out of a sense of community and personal beliefs. Give me a break! Obviously, the Do-gooders don't go into that kind of work for the money—although they are making a better living than the people they "serve"—and even though the words are about supporting and serving, they're basically trying to fill their own needs, to use the jargon. . . . When you're disabled and these Do-gooders pull their shit, there is allegedly nothing that you can do. I know. I've suffered years of the Do-gooders' afflictions. Their game is about wanting to be in control of other peoples' lives. (1994:165–168)[3]

In a review of David Hevey's *The Creatures Time Forgot*, which, among other things, examines charity advertising, the feminist and disability rights activist Anne Finger makes a similar point about charity:

Hevey points out that charities function to "bind up the wounds of society"; that their raison d'être is to work for amelioration of such wounds rather than for fundamental social change that would prevent such wounds in the first place; most importantly, that in locating the oppression in the impairment itself (that is, in the body or mind of the disabled person) rather than in the social organizations that actively exclude and oppress disabled people (from the state on down to the family), charities, by their very nature, turn away from social and political change and toward the individual "help the handicapped" solutions. Not only does the charity industry as a whole function this way under capitalism (and what a relief it is to read a book about disability that isn't scared of naming capitalism as a source of our oppression!) but each individual charity must compete with other charities for the "charitable dollar." Thus, charity advertising aims at simultaneously creating an image of "its" disease or impairment and of that particular charity as the custodian/savior/earthly representative of all those with that dreaded impairment. (1993:29–31)

Hevey, putting Gramsci's notion of hegemony to good use, argues that charities are the principal institution in controlling people with disabilities. Laura Hershey, a journalist and disability rights activist, perfectly portrayed charity advertising and the DRM's response:

Photo one: a woman's eyes are covered by a blindfold. She's bound up in ropes, chains, and barbed wire. Photo two: a different woman stands, slouching—again, her arms and torso are wrapped in layers of rope and chain. These black and white photos don't advertise an X-rated film; they're actually a plea for sympathy. Commissioned by the National Muscular Sclerosis Society—ostensibly to dramatize the unpredictable symptoms of MS— these advertisements began appearing in media markets throughout the country. With their violent, pseudopornographic images, the ads reinforce stereotypes about both gender and disability, perpetuating the notion that a woman with a disability is naturally, unescapably helpless—the perfect victim. . . . As a woman disabled by a neuromuscular condition, and as a feminist . . . I've joined in protesting comedian Jerry Lewis' sideshow, the MDA Labor Day telethon, which uses sex role stereotypes and sappy music to convey the "devastating terrible" effects of neuromuscular disabilities—and thus to evoke pity....("This is a kid who won't be asked to the prom," laments one girl's father.) (1995:96)

Although Golfus, Finger, and Hershey live in the United States and Hevey lives in England, their assessments mirror those of activists who live in the periphery.

Alexander Phiri: "It's interesting that when we got started, the rehabilitation industry tried to destroy us. They told the government that we were part of the guerrilla movement at that time. This could have created very difficult problems for us. The white government could have crushed us.... I know about these charities firsthand. When I passed through primary school and passed the placement tests I wanted to go to secondary school, but the charity institution where I lived said I couldn't go. There were two of us who had done well and had applied to a mission school [secondary school]. The institution said I should forget school and become a cobbler. They had these ideas about disabled people only being able to get by with craft work. During all these years, no matter how successful I was in school, I was always discouraged. The Jauros Jiri institution offered me a secretarial job, and when I refused, people there told me this was the only job I would ever be offered. . . . The role of charities is to help us by controlling us, not liberating us from all that holds us down."

Friday Mandla Mavuso: "Many people in social service agencies saw our Committee as ungratefuls and especially the Crippled Care Association saw us as threatening."

Rosangela Berman Bieler: "When we were organizing at the rehab center, we began to put out newsletters such as . . . *Clandestino.* . . . It was because of this newsletter that the rehab center kicked us out."

These experiences and conclusions should not be surprising. The mission of charities is to take care of people who are permanently outside society's channels of livelihood, or who, given particular conditions, might rebel. As far back as 1916, Henry Ford sent social workers into his workers' communities to assist in their "organization" (Harvey 1992:126). Social workers are the one segment of traditional social services that could play a progressive role by teaching people how to become independent, but they usually (there are exceptions) follow agency procedures, as well as their own helping predispositions, and try to take care of their "clients." This is what Paulo Freire meant when he said the moment social workers eschewed education for "assistencialism," they became "facilitators of paternalism, dependency" (1987:115). Some nation-states are so poor that charities have few resources and little impact. In other places charities are a major social institution. In both cases, on whatever level of social intervention these institutions and networks of institutions operate, they control under the auspices of helping the helpless and are salient factors in the lives of persons with disabilities. They also make it possible for others to avoid the responsibility to provide access for everyone. People with disabilities are told, "Go to so and so. It is a special program just for the handicapped."

Charities and traditional social services satisfy their role as controller in different ways. First, they take responsibility for (take responsibility away from) people. If this is resisted, they engage in degradation ("You will never amount to anything, you should be grateful"). Next, they separate and target dissenters (ungratefuls), especially politically minded

ones, and move with dispatch and impunity to crush them when necessary. For the most part charities are not staffed by evil, manipulative people. Charities react this way because they live off the economic and psychological dependence of people with disabilities. What is needed are
programs and institutions that support people in their quest for independence and respect, not operate to maintain the existing relations of
domination and subordination.

The Hierarchy of Disability

---

*In China, there is nothing for those with mental disabilities.
I would say people with cerebral palsy are in the same group
because they are mistakenly lumped in with mental
retardation. These people are brutally treated. Their
condition makes ours [people who are blind] seem tolerable.*
          Charles Leung, chair, Supervisory Committee,
          Hong Kong Federation of Handicapped Youth

There is a hierarchy of disability. This hierarchy extends
across continents and zones of economic development. It breaks down
like this: people with mental disabilities and those perceived as having
mental disabilities have the most difficult lives, followed by people with
hearing disabilities. People with physical and visual disabilities have
greater political, social, and economic opportunities and support systems.

Why is this? First, it is noteworthy that people who are blind have had
the longest-established social services and, conversely, people with hearing and mental disabilities the shortest. Second, mental disabilities are
not visible, which contributes to isolation and inadequate support systems. Third, people who are mentally ill have the least capacity to organize their lives and fight for their rights. Also, people who are mentally
ill are commonly abused and even hated because many people fear that
"crazy people" will do something crazy (to them). Fourth, the appropriate support systems for people with mental and hearing disabilities
are the most complex and necessarily professionalized and technical.

In many parts of Latin America and Africa, women with mental illness are victims of harassment and rape. Men are often savagely beaten,
sometimes dressed up as clowns and made a public spectacle. Ultimately,
one way or another, they disappear and perish. Families know this to be
the case and not infrequently kill children with mental disabilities—as a

favor. Most often, the mentally ill are institutionalized or abandoned to live as homeless beggars.

Francisco Rodriguez: "I would say that disability in Mexico breaks down along four categories in terms of services and attitudes. The most marginalized people with disabilities in Mexico are people with mental deficiencies. These people have the most problems. Although there are a few expensive institutions, most people do not have any access to psychological support. There is virtually no family or individual counseling for people with mental disabilities. The second most marginalized group of people with disabilities are people who are deaf. You need to understand that we have very few skilled interpreters in the whole country of Mexico. This makes it very difficult to provide education to people who need these support services and is an impossible barrier for communication in everyday activities. The other two groups of people with disabilities [blind and mobility impaired] are much better organized and have many more services than the first two groups, although it is fair to say services for us are lacking as well."

Alexander Phiri: "I would say the blind and physically disabled have the best chances, although the chances for us are poor. For the deaf and mentally disabled, I see no hope in the short run unless they come from rich families."

Danilo Delfin: "I believe people with mental retardation are treated the worst. In the Philippines, people say the mentally retarded are unlucky. There are growing numbers of people working with or for physically disabled, although I think the blind are the most politically conscious, especially in Vietnam, the Philippines, and Thailand. In Cambodia only the amputees are finding services."

Orlando Perez: "[In Nicaragua] I think people with orthopedic disabilities have made the most progress. At one time, the blind had more possibilities. People with other disabilities have great difficulties in Central America."

Maria da Comceição Caussat: "[In Brazil] even within these groups, there are wide differences based on what kind of disability one has. For example, deaf people have almost no possibility to go to school. Blind people are better treated and receive more education. People with cerebral palsy are treated incredibly bad, worse than other people with physical disabilities. In fact, they are treated like people with mental retardation. Outside of these folks [the blind], physically disabled have the best chances for jobs and education."

Any explanation of the way in which each "category" in this hierarchy, however arbitrary, affects the experience of disability oppression would require its own chapter. Suffice it to say here that these differences are significant and complex. For instance, people often have multiple disabilities that cut across simple categories (this is particularly true of elderly persons) or have disabilities (as disparate as chronic fatigue syndrome and AIDS) that are poorly understood. For the disability rights movement, this complex hierarchy presents a variety of issues and histories, and, in its practice, organizational and programmatic problems it has not fully solved.

Violence and Disability

*I suffered until I was thirteen years old. Then my life
changed. I became friends with a man who offered to help me.
He was the answer to my dreams because I was so tired of
living in poverty, so tired of suffering. I thanked God for the
opportunity to end my misery. The first thing my friend did
was to put me to the test. He gave me a package that weighed
three and a half kilograms. He also gave me a .45 revolver.
He warned me that in no case was I to lose the package; that
my future depended on getting it to Mexicali. The package
reached its destination, and when I returned, my friend was
waiting for me. Not until then did I realize that the package
I had delivered contained cocaine. "You've passed the test,"
my friend told me. "Do you want to keep working for
me?" . . . When my daughter turned two years old, I decided
to throw her a party, never imagining that it could be
dangerous. I had her in my arms when a pickup arrived and
several men started shooting at us. The first shots hit my wife
and killed her instantly; then they hit me. With seven bullets
inside me, I watched them kill my daughter. Then everything
went blank, one of the bullets passed through my spine,
paralyzing my lower body.*

> Anonymous leader of Projecto Proximo, in
> Hesperian Foundation, "Newsletter from the Sierra
> Madre #25"

Just as there are relationships among political economy, culture, and disability that inform why and how people are isolated and invisible, unable to obtain needed support and equipment, and subjected to intense stratification, there too is a relationship among these that gives rise to an extraordinary level of violence. People with disabilities may be the group that is most vulnerable to violence because such an unusually high percentage live and work in the streets.

Violence is not only a common cause of disability, it is also a source of fear after one becomes disabled. When I was in Nicaragua in 1985, Gladys Baez, one of the Sandinista revolution's most respected leaders and a victim of years of torture, spoke about the psychological devastation people, especially children, had undergone as a result of sustaining disabilities during the repression of the Somoza dictatorship.[4] Violence creates fear in people no matter how directed or random it is. Judy Panko Reis, the administrator of Chicago's Health Clinic for Women with Disabilities, sustained a traumatic brain injury during an attack she and her fiancé suffered in Hawaii where they were vacationing.

Judy Panko Reis: "We went camping at the state park on the Big Island. There we were brutally attacked and Philip died. I had a pulverized skull and was left for dead. That's how I sustained the injury in the right hemisphere of my brain. For many years I had a hard time getting out of that tent. For a while I wished I hadn't lived. I lived in chronic depression, which you don't even realize until you are coming out of it. It was always there, nightmares and phobias about the man I later married and our kid. I was always afraid that they would be killed or taken away."

Violence has many facets: political repression, personal retaliation, environmental and spatial, chance. Violence is rampant throughout the world, although violence in Western Europe pales in comparison to the Third World, the United States, and Eastern Europe. For example, in Chicago, gunshot wounds recently passed driving and diving accidents as the number one reason for spinal cord injuries. While endemic violence is blind to its many victims, it is not simply a product of people with a predisposition to violence. It is a logical outcome of a world in which many people are wealthy and powerful and use violence to protect that wealth and power and in which many more people believe they must resort to violence to survive. A visit to any of the Third World's urban centers will expose the stark brutality of this logic.

For example, Johannesburg, South Africa's largest city, is considered by many to be the most dangerous city in the world. It is surrounded by some of the largest townships in the world, one of which, Soweto, with 2 million people, is more than twice Johannesburg's size.[5] The struggle to survive in Soweto and the many other townships surrounding South Africa's major cities inevitably spills over into the already intense city boundaries. When desperate poverty exists so close to colossal wealth, the consequences are predictable.

This is also apparent in Rio de Janeiro, where the luxurious boroughs of Ipanema, Lablon, and parts of Copacabana are nestled next to some of the most densely populated slums (*favelas*) in the world. While Brazil's economic miracle of the 1970s was creating some of the wealthiest people in the world (mainly those in and connected to the military dictatorship that ran the country for decades), it was also magnifying the country's contrast between rich and poor. The consequences again are predictable. A murder wave pushed the number of homicides in Rio to five hundred for one month in 1988, a rate that would give Rio three times as many killings per year as New York City, which is roughly the same size. Most urban violence is horizontal (poor against poor) or institutional (killing by police/death squads/gangs) in nature. Thousands of homeless children are murdered every year in each of the major cities of Brazil.[6] The illegal drug industry is only the largest of the criminal activities in which people are engaged to survive and, in a few cases, prosper. For example, I was told by Rosangela Berman Bieler that one hundred cars are stolen every day in Rio. A culture of violence has evolved throughout Latin America, Africa, and part of Asia which imperils everyday life for millions of people with disabilities.

Paulo Saturnino Figueiredo: "The Brazilian culture is now rooted in extreme violence. It results from a super-concentration of income and a super-concentration of image. This kind of culture has a high possibility of making and discarding disabled people."

Danilo Delfin: "The political culture in Kampuchea is 'see no evil, speak no evil.' When we went into Kampuchea to organize for disability-related legislation, people were afraid to get involved because they might get disappeared for participation. The only way is through international organizations, which will ironically make the law's implementation even harder."

To the extent that violence is a product of poverty and powerlessness, it is not surprising that many acts of violence are overtly political. This is particularly relevant here because political people with disabilities are easy targets of repression. In the Philippines, Kampuchea, and El Salvador, where there has been military and/or political stalemate, the issues of political violence and disability are extremely complicated. Personal security is paramount. In November 1992, Felipe Barrera, a disabled soldier of El Salvador's revolutionary army, made a speaking tour of the United States to raise funds for badly needed supplies and equipment for others disabled in the decade-long war. He highlighted the complexity of reintegration for disabled members of the Farabundo Martí Liberación Nacional (FMLN), the guerrilla wing of five political opposition groups in El Salvador.

Felipe Barrera: "One of the elements that many people with disabilities are affected by is the question of reunification of war veterans of the FMLN. You have to remember, disabled veterans have been underground, some of us for eight or ten years, so we have been totally separated from our communities and families. Another big issue for us is personal security. Many of us have great fear coming back from Cuba or from underground with the prospect of intimidation or violence from the Salvadoran security forces or death squads. We are so obvious because of our disabilities."

Danilo Delfin expressed a similar message as it concerns Southeast Asia, especially Kampuchea, where the Khmer Rouge have fought a war of extermination for decades.

Danilo Delfin: "Cambodia has been fighting more than thirty years, since they were children, so their attitudes are conditioned by this experience. If you are disabled, you automatically have people after you. The Khmer Rouge think you were a government soldier, and the military assumes you were a guerrilla. It is very dangerous for people with disabilities, especially in the refugee camps."

Inaccessibility, Space, and the Environment

My school years were very hard. There was a rumor around school that if you touched my wheelchair you would become paralyzed. So it was initially very hard to get other students to help me which would of been nice because the school wasn't accessible, including the cafeteria and the bathroom. The school officials always maintained they could not make these areas accessible because they were unable to pay for it.

Alexander Phiri, chairperson, NCDP2

A wheelchair user, I am always asked on returning from a trip what the accessibility was like. My reply is always the same: "It isn't good." Of course, the meaning of "accessibility" varies depending on where you are and what you consider access to encompass. In Bali, the entrance to every house is an archway of steps designed to keep the evil spirits away. The rubble of wartorn countries like the former Yugoslavia, Chechnya, Kampuchea, Angola, or El Salvador is not hospitable for either mobility or communication. Europe's Old World architecture may be quaint, but it is certainly not conducive to significant rehabilitation. Urban America (both North and South) has greater access than do the rural areas because of the greater availability of taxis, public buildings, restaurants, stores, apartments, schools, and so on. But, as I shall describe, there still is a long way to go in achieving barrier-free environments.

Most important, accessibility means different things to different people. For me, it includes something that is less tangible than architecture and communication devices. It is the likelihood of receiving the support, services, and devices necessary for a reasonable quality of life. It involves the totality of life for people with disabilities. Access is then a social construct, not simply an architectural one. For example, it does not help to make a building accessible if people with mobility disabilities cannot get to the building because of street or transportation or attitudinal barriers. Likewise, it does little good to make one subway station barrier-free if there are not other accessible stations. That transportation, health care, equipment, and programs are found only in cities introduces the question of how rural people can manage to survive.

Fernando Rodriguez: "It is important to note in understanding the context of disability in Mexico that while we have excellent hospitals and rehabilitation centers, there are only a few of these; and they are concentrated in the most important urban areas. Outside of these sites, only outpatient therapy is available unless you are rich and can afford a personal therapist, so people with disabilities have virtually no access to health care."

Access is a simple proposition obscured by prejudice that prioritizes projects and resources in terms of tradition and wealth. What generates more wealth is undertaken; what does not, is not. Alexander Phiri's comments above demonstrate how insidious backward attitudes are, especially in combination with a perceived scarcity of resources.

Appropriate housing is another necessity that people with disabilities typically go without. This renders a forceful connection between political economy and accessibility. It illustrates the austere differences between development and underdevelopment. For most people in peripheral economic zones, housing means a small space occupied by many people. Notwithstanding the significant number of those who are abandoned, most people with disabilities live with family members in small houses, shacks, or shelters. Most have running water and electricity but not necessarily drainage. Family members share eating and sleeping space in these quarters.

Friday Mandla Mavuso: "Of course it was very difficult to survive in a township. People live in houses that are four meters wide, and the toilet is outside. There may be up to fifteen people in some of these houses. You have a bedroom and a kitchen and maybe a sitting room. At night, everybody sleeps everywhere. . . . Many people are rejected after they incur a disability and when they come home because they cannot, or people think they cannot, be responsible to help the family survive. Many people I know who use wheelchairs are just shocked by the physical accommodation issues."

Housing in the Third World is likely not to be accessible for people who use mobility devices like wheelchairs, braces, and crutches. Accessible bathrooms are rare, so people with mobility disabilities require assistance. A physically disabled person is often given a place—perhaps on the porch or in the living room—where he or she will remain during the day. A few necessary things, like water, a urine bottle, or a snack, are left close by. These conditions dominate the residential landscape throughout the Third World.

Affordable, accessible housing is not readily available in the United States. Many people with disabilities, possibly most, must adjust to living in places that do not afford practical and functional access. Houses and apartments have steps, narrow doorways, unreachable toilets and showers, and hard-to-use counters and utilities and lack sound and light devices for those with sensory disabilities, and so forth. These handicaps add up to a loss of control in one's everyday life.

Everyone I interviewed reported that housing, schools, stores and markets, and public buildings are for the most part inaccessible. This is the case in the most modern urban areas. There are, of course, gradations of inaccessibility. Some places are easier to get around in than others. Most larger cities have curb-cut some of the major streets, taxis are readily available (although many people with disabilities cannot afford them), many public buildings have elevators (although some of these have entrance steps), and many restaurants and bars are accessible. Where these are not available, people with disabilities often become quite creative. They must be creative, or they are stuck somewhere, out of sight. For example, driveways are used as ramps; bystanders are asked for assistance up steps; people crawl up bus steps; and friends show people who have visual disabilities ways to get around.

Whether one can get into stores, shops, and markets is one more area that dramatically divides developed and underdeveloped economic regions. In the United States and Europe, shopping malls and large supermarkets, where many products are easily found, are usually accessible. Drive-through fast-food outlets, banking, and pharmacies and ordering via computers, television, and catalogs further enhance easy access to needed products. Access to food and other products may be more difficult in rural communities, but only relatively so. Transportation is crucial in either case. In the United States and Europe, transportation has been a long-standing problem.

Rachel Hurst: "There has been nothing in the way of transportation options here. It's dreadful. People are stuck or dependent on others to take them around. Indeed, I think transportation is the key link to all other aspects of life. It's crucial."

Most of Europe is far behind the United States, where limited transportation options appeared only in the last fifteen years. Only in northern Europe, where main-line public buses and trains continue to be inaccessible, are paratransit (door-to-door, dial-a-ride) vans widely available. Paradoxically, while paratransit vans fill a crucial void, they segregate people with mobility limitations, contributing to what Edward Said (following Fanon) emphasizes as a crucial dimension to oppression: segregated or "sequestered" space (Said 1993:326–333).

Mike Ervin: "Dial-a-Ride is ridiculously degrading. When it first came, my hopes were raised, but the experience of calling the day before at six in the morning, being told no, or having to wait for the minivans to show up and then riding around by myself in these 'special' vans was too much to take."

Adolph Ratzka: "While it is good that paratransit vans are readily available, it, like a lot of our other services, puts people to sleep. They don't recognize segregated transportation reinforces the stereotypes about us as sick or special."

Rachel Hurst: "The abundance of those [paratransit] services [in Sweden] may get people around, but it sends all the wrong messages, that people with disabilities are helpless."

The greatest advances in transportation have been made in the United States. Many cities have both main-line access and paratransit services (although these are often limited). Although the Americans with Disabilities Act of 1992 mandates that all newly purchased intracity buses and a minimum number of "key" train stations be accessible, huge problems remain. The only accessible rapid rail systems are the Bay Area Rapid Transit and Washington, D.C.'s system. In Chicago, less than 25 percent of stations are accessible. Boston, New York, and Philadelphia are even worse.

Accessing public and semipublic transportation within and between Third World cities is incredibly difficult, although very inexpensive. There is often no room for people with disabilities on these buses, minivans (private jitney-type operations), and trucks. Transportation for poor people in the Third World often resembles hitchhiking. One waits for a minivan or truck to come by, flags it down, jumps on, and pays a small fee. These vehicles are always packed. Standing room only means room only for those who can stand for long periods.

Access is affected by other kinds of geographic considerations. In many parts of the world people must travel by boat. Images of jammed transport boats going up the Amazon or down the Niger or Yangtze River are common in *National Geographic* or the *New York Times* travel section. Needless to say, these means of transportation are out of the question for a person with a physical disability. It can get more complicated. The geographic, political, and ethnic diversity of a country like Indonesia, which has thirteen thousand islands, hundreds of cultures, and a fascist political system, presents insurmountable travel barriers to the vast majority of people with disabilities.

Mobility in Asia is mind-boggling given the small spaces and large numbers of people. China alone has more than one-fourth of the world's population, in a space comparable to the continental United States. Indonesia is just as densely populated. In all my travels, Bangkok, where 40 percent of the Thai people live, is the hardest city to get around. Although the actual structural inaccessibility (lack of ramps, curb cuts, elevators) is more or less the same throughout the Third World, the streets in Bangkok are almost impossible to cross. Whereas in other cities (even in the giants São Paulo, Santiago, and Buenos Aires) I have often used the streets, this is too dangerous in Bangkok. During traffic gridlock, which is almost perpetual, motorcyclists, in the hundreds of thousands, use the sidewalks. Bangkok is a wheelchair user's worst nightmare. Jakarta and Bombay are close runners-up.

Space is a critical component of accessibility. Space is experienced differently by different people in different places. As Claude Lévi-Strauss wrote in *Tristes Tropiques,* space "has its own values, just as sounds and perfumes have their own colours, and feelings weight" ([1955] 1992:123). A Polish writer once wrote a book after he had a stroke. I cannot remember the writer's name, but I do remember that he argued that space for children seems to expand whereas for adults it seems to shrink. The wide-eyed possibility of youth withers with age. Following his stroke, this writer had discovered something quite interesting about space. He maintained that for children space actually expands horizontally; for older people it expands vertically. He had begun to notice steps he had obliviously traversed many times—the slight incline in the street in front of his house, the upper and lower sections of the neighborhood park, and so forth. He attributed this to age, but more accurately his age and stroke translated into a mobility limitation. Disability indeed expands one's perception of space.

By now I hope it is apparent that accessibility is contingent on the environment itself. As the environment is destroyed, accessibility is negatively affected. Air pollution is just the most obvious example: people with respiratory disabilities, chronic fatigue syndrome, allergies, and chemical sensitivities are acutely restricted. This is sharply put in a resolution passed by disability rights activists at the UN International Symposium on Environment and Disability in 1992: "Persons with disabilities are keenly observant of the disabling consequences to nature and humans alike: Air and water pollution and the disposal of toxic waste; Poverty and malnutrition; Militarization and war; Lack of regulation of transnational corporations; Human genetic engineering and intolerance of biodiversity; Climate change which contributes to disabling environments such as deserts or flooded areas" (UN 1992).

URBAN VERSUS RURAL AREAS

There are differences in opportunities, access, and attitudes for people with disabilities between the cities and the rural areas. There is more marginalization and poverty [in the countryside]. There are often no streets, just houses. The rural culture is very different. The people are more timid. At the sight of someone who cannot walk, people think we are sick. The idea is often that disability is connected to sin. Further, people with disabilities are very isolated and hard to organize

*in the rural areas. It is common that people with disabilities
stay in the house and never leave.*

Cornelio Nuñez Ordaz, president, Wheelchair
Sports Association of Oaxaca, Mexico

It is apparent that more enlightened attitudes and greater
opportunities reside in zones of advanced economic development than
in the Third World. It is also apparent that these same advantages are
relatively more available in the periphery's urban centers than in its rural
areas.

Individual rural residences or compounds in the periphery appear to
be where the most privation and isolation occur. These sites establish
one end of a spectrum that moves from villages to small and medium-
sized cities to the mega-metropolis. Paradoxically, villages and small
towns seem to be the only places where people can hope to receive family and community support in obtaining shelter and food. In these communities, though, there is no hope for a decent education, any real independence, or any work. People with disabilities may not disappear in
villages as they do in isolated rural areas, but they are stuck in dependence and only the most tenacious ones escape.

Cornelio Nuñez Ordaz: "I was born in a small village called La Blanco
Zucitan in 1954. I had polio before I was one. I grew up walking with my
hands. I lived on the floor, on the ground. My family was large, with ten
kids. My father built a cart for me when I got older. It was like a wheelbar-
row. My older brother helped me beginning when he was nine, but other
children laughed at him. I was the only one in the village to contract polio.
While my parents were illiterate, they were open-minded about my disability. It was difficult for them because many people thought my disability was
from malnutrition or from 'castilo devino' [a curse]. The doctors assured
my family it was a medical problem, but it was very difficult to get medical
treatments because we had no money. I helped milk the cows and worked
with the pigs and chickens. At fifteen, I was using a cart pulled by goats but
I soon went back to walking around with my hands because many kids in
town ran away from me when they saw the goats, especially girls. . . . At
twenty, a friend of mine suggested I move to Oaxaca City and get a wheelchair. When I brought this up with my family, my parents were worried
about me surviving in Oaxaca. They said people would not help me and
that there were many cars and that I might get run over. I insisted. So in
1974, my father gave me about $160 (U.S.) and I left for Oaxaca by bus.
As soon as I arrived I went to the Governor's office and asked to see the
wife of the Governor who was at the time the President of the Rehabilitation Center of Oaxaca. At first they said that it was not possible to see this

woman. But I was very determined and never left. Finally, after waiting there for a long time, I got my first wheelchair."

People tend to become absorbed into the labyrinth of the larger cities and disappear in a different way. Third World cities are stark microcosms of the paradoxical realities of underdevelopment. Here, great concentrations of wealth stare obliquely into the faces of desperate people, obscured by a general resignation as the city's infrastructure collapses and gridlock frustrates people's mobility. The ever-present throng creates anonymity and loneliness.

There are ironies concerning accessibility that are informed by the differences between urban and rural areas. Generally, in the developed world the farther one moves from the central city, the easier it is to get around. But consider the terrain in the barrios, favelas, and slums that ring metropolitan centers in the periphery such as Mexico City (e.g., Nezahualcoyotl), Rio de Janeiro (Rocinho), Lima (Villa El Salvador), and Caracas (Ranchos). I only name a few in Latin America because I am the most familiar with these. Some of these slums perch on hillsides without concrete streets or sidewalks (as in Rio), some are set on barren land (as in Mexico City) without city services as simple as electricity, water, or garbage collection. Smokey Mountain, the biggest slum in Manila, is located on a garbage dump site, as is a slum in San Salvador. Some people say the slums outside Cairo are the largest in the world. The best-known slum in Thailand is located in a backwater off Bangkok's terribly polluted canals. These places, considered by people with money to be uninhabitable, present a prohibitive combination of incredible population density and impassable terrain for the vast number of people with disabilities living in them.

The most striking differences between city and countryside may be in terms of attitudes about disability. There are changing beliefs about and toward disability in the world, but these changes have been slower in rural areas.[7] That some change *is* taking place in the countryside is noteworthy. This is a product of the marginal modernization of the countryside in some regions, the impact of Western culture and images throughout the periphery, out-migration to the developed world by people who continue their ties to their home communities, and, most important, the impact of the disability rights movement within these regions.

Michael Masutha: "I cannot speak about the entire country. Even in Soweto, you find a rural setting in an urban context. You still find people in rural areas who are self-subsistence farming, have little or no education and transportation, and believe in witchcraft. On the other hand, you find an emergence of a Western generation. Even in the rural areas, some youth have had the opportunity to study in urban areas, and when they return they bring their music, clothing, and so on."

Alexander Phiri: "I think the attitudes in the rural areas are the worst. These areas have very entrenched ideas that are very bad, that lead to treating disabled people always like children or worse. We are connected to evil because of rural peoples' notions of witchcraft."

Rajendra Vyas: "I don't believe there are regional differences when it comes to attitudes toward disability, but there are differences between cities and villages. Hindus believe in Karma. They believe I am blind today because of past misdeeds. I don't think this is strictly believed today in cities, but definitely in the villages."

Panomwan Bootem: "People in Thailand laugh at the deaf, especially when we are signing. We have an advantage in the cities because we get training in communication, but in the rural areas children who are deaf are kept at home."

Wiriya Namsiripongpun: "If a rural family in Thailand allows a person with a disability to work, it looks like the family is failing in its responsibilities."

Federico Fleischmann: "In the rural areas, it is different. If a boy or girl is born with a disability, I don't know if the family feels guilty or punished or whatever, but they really feel that this is not a problem to be solved. They prefer to ignore the child—especially fathers, not so much mothers. Especially in the rural areas, fathers are very ashamed. Mothers would take care or try to take care, but it is still difficult for the child."

Gabriella Brimmer: "In the rural areas, the process of rehabilitation is more difficult. If they [disabled people] have the economic means, they can be taken to the nearest rehabilitation center; and if not, they will be cared for until they die."

Fadila Lagadien: "Attitudes are a big barrier, especially in the rural areas. I have known families who have rejected their own kind because of a disability because they thought it was because of God or some omen. In a rural area children with polio are even hidden because of these attitudes. People who become disabled when they are adults do not have to deal with this particular attitude."

While the gap between rural and urban attitudes is an important ideological factor of everyday life in the Third World, it should not be overstated. Urban attitudes are not that enlightened. We need to look no farther than the United States to see that while attitudes toward disability are less imbued with superstition and contempt, they are still backward.

Chronicling Everyday Life in a Complex World

Chronicling everyday life in a world fragmented by economic zones and thousands of cultures and unified, even compressed, by invisible economic laws and cyberoptics requires great caution and produces generalizations that endanger the realities of individual lived experience. The features of everyday life presented in this chapter are prominent in the lives of the vast majority of people with disabilities. I can say this with great confidence based on direct as well as indirect experience. What particularizes and differentiates one's experiences has to do with how survival or "struggle of life" is understood. There is an ongoing struggle everywhere for most people with disabilities.

PART III

Empowerment and Organization

When I was young, for example, it was an insult to be called black. The blacks have now taken over this once pejorative term and made of it a rallying cry and a badge of honor and are teaching their children to be proud that they are black. . . . To be liberated from the stigma of blackness by embracing it is to cease, for ever, one's interior agreement and collaboration with the author of one's degradation.

James Baldwin, No Name in the Street

CHAPTER 7

Empowered Consciousness and the Philosophy of Empowerment

The experiences related by disability rights activists throughout this book speak of the impossible, accidents of fortune, catharsis, transformation, radicalization, and conversion. They illustrate the powerful role of consciousness when, as Tracy Chapman sings in "Why," "the blind remove their blinders and the speechless speak the truth." They also show how, out of similar and divergent experiences, people with disabilities have acquired a consciousness of themselves and the world around them. This new understanding has affected their aspirations and responsibilities. They have come to a *raised* consciousness of themselves not only as people with disabilities but also as oppressed people. Moreover, they have become political activists because through their *raised* consciousness they have become *empowered*. They no longer think of disability as a medical condition but as a human condition. They are no longer interested in the "welfare of the handicapped"; they are interested in the human rights of people with disabilities. They have joined a liberation movement to free people with disabilities from political, economic, and cultural oppression.

In *Femininity and Domination,* Sandra Bartky describes the power of raised consciousness:

This experience, the acquiring of a "raised" consciousness, in spite of its disturbing aspects, is an immeasurable advance over that false consciousness which it replaces. The scales fall from our eyes. We are no longer required to struggle against unreal enemies, to put others' interests ahead of our own, or to hate ourselves. We begin to understand why we have such depreciated images of ourselves and why so many of us are lacking any genuine conviction of personal worth. Understanding, even beginning to understand this, makes it possible to change. Coming to see things differently, we are able to make out possibilities for liberating collective action and for unprecedented personal growth, possibilities which a deceptive sexist social reality had heretofore concealed. No longer do we have to practice upon ourselves that mutilation of intellect and personality required of individuals who, caught up in an irrational and destructive system, are nevertheless not allowed to regard it as anything but sane, progressive, and normal. Moreover, that feeling of alienation from established society which is so prominent a feature of feminist experience may be counterbalanced by a new identification with women of all conditions and a growing sense of solidarity with other feminist consciousness, in spite of its ambiguities, confusions, and trials, is apprehended by those in whom it develops as an experience of liberation. (1990:27)

It is not possible to definitively explain the changes Bartky describes. There will never be *a* or *the* definitive proof of why an individual attains raised consciousness. People are too unique and consciousness too complex. Many philosophers have tried, with mixed results.[1] The best I can do is provide a synthesis of experiences, stories, and anecdotes from the disability rights activists I interviewed. While their experiences encompass a limited array of disabilities, cultures, and institutions, they are compelling and revealing. The influences of family and class, school, poverty and injustice, war and violence, and chance are acutely evident. In each of these cases, creative and clever people figured out the *ways of everyday life*. One example perfectly illustrates this point. Twenty years ago in Zimbabwe, a group of young men with disabilities, institutionalized in a Jauros Jiri residential facility and self-described "inmates," came to the astounding conclusion that the only way to make a better place for themselves was to organize.

Ranga Mupindu: "We began to organize strikes and demonstrations. We started our organization within the institution, it really scared the institution's authorities. . . . We also set up a scam, to pay for our organizing efforts. You know, many people gave donations to Jauros Jiri, but they were never passed on to us, so we called together this group of criminals who were living close to the institution and we told them that we would get these donations to them so they could sell them on the black market if we got half. They thought we were cool to call on them so we made a deal. This scam lasted two years. It was a lucrative deal for us and helped us get paper, supplies, and so forth. When we were discovered, I was dismissed."

Empowered consciousness is essential for political activists. Without a conscious interest in everyday life, social change is subject to whimsy and chance. If social progress takes place only by the force of time or by chance, there is little reason to be a political organizer. The only way to empowerment is through the conscious activity of people themselves. This is one lesson that all oppressed groups have had to learn.

Toward an Understanding of Empowered Consciousness

I called the independent living center in Chicago and they put me in touch with a number of disabled suburban women who were organizing a meeting around transportation. The first meeting I went to I was totally intimidated. I kept thinking throughout the meeting that I am not like these people and they are not like me. I'm a businesswoman. But there quickly began an amazing shift in my consciousness. We decided to start going to the public transit board meetings and organizing protests. Once we started meeting with the professionals at that agency, I felt in my element, except immediately I was categorized as "you people." What do "you people" want? we were asked. So that radicalized me. That was, you might say, the greening of Judy Panko Reis. My businesswoman view was collapsing. I started realizing the people I was with were more like me than anybody else. . . . Unless I had become pissed off at my condition and gotten into transportation advocacy when I had, I may have never recognized my own self.

> Judy Panko Reis, administrative director, Chicago
> Health Clinic for Women with Disabilities

In 1981, I was invited to go to Singapore to the Disabled Peoples' International conference, representing the Philippine National Commission of the Disabled. That one event changed my life. I went there to have some fun and get a free trip but as soon as I got there I became involved in all these controversies about how disabled people could take control of their lives. I remember seeing Ed Roberts and thinking that if a man with the disability he had could do so much, I could do something, too. This was the first time I had met activists from anywhere outside the Philippines. When I returned, I was committed to organizing.

> Danilo Delfin, regional development officer,
> Disabled Peoples' International

Because I was having problems with mobility, I started using a wheelchair in 1975. I saw the wheelchair as a wonderful

mobility aid that would allow me to continue my work. I was
immediately struck by peoples' reactions. I can say my
consciousness was raised almost overnight. I was teaching
dance and drama at the time. It was so strange because I felt
the same the day before I started using the wheelchair as the
day I started using the wheelchair, but I was immediately
labeled incapable. I decided I had to do something. I quickly
realized that a single person never gets anywhere so I tried to
figure out how I could do something collectively.

> Rachel Hurst, project director, Disability Awareness
> in Action, London, England

The lives of disability rights activists reveal a lot about raised consciousness. "Raised consciousness" is shown as an experientially evolved awareness of self. Most often, raised consciousness involves a change in consciousness whereby the (false) notion of disability as a pitiful, medical condition has been replaced by the (true) awareness of disability as a social condition. This new consciousness is profoundly liberating. It allows individuals to recognize themselves in the context of something bigger than themselves and enables them to appreciate the commonalities they have with others. Isolation and estrangement are replaced by association and connection.

Although their consciousness about themselves and their identity may differ, these people have departed significantly from the values of the dominant culture. The continuum of raised consciousness defies the dominant images and meanings of disability; it is resistant.

The term "raised consciousness" may be misleading. It is used to signify a movement or turn away from the dominant ideology that emasculates people's sense of self and distorts their sense of identity. It is not higher or deeper, it is more authentic and organic than false consciousness, which is contrived, or, to use Noam Chomsky's term, manufactured. By raised consciousness I do not mean a unified, politically correct consciousness. It is a continuum of changing values and ideas that rejects domination. It is in this sense a process, what Paulo Freire and Kwame Nkrumah have referred to as "conscientization."

Some writers have called the consciousness of oppressed people about their own culture and their own identity "borderland consciousness." The border metaphor is fitting because of the complex, conflictual, and peripheral experiences of "minorities" (those outside dominant culture). Peter McLaren calls border identity "not simply an identity that is anticapitalist and counterhegemonic but . . . critically utopian" (1994:66).

In illustrating this oppositional consciousness, McLaren directs us to Chandra Talpade Mohanty, who describes *mestiza* consciousness as "a consciousness of the borderlands, a consciousness born of the historical collusion of Anglo and Mexican cultures and frames of reference. It is a plural consciousness in that it requires understanding multiple, often opposing ideas and knowledges and negotiating these knowledges, not just taking a simple counterstance" (1991:35).

For political activists, including the disability rights activists I interviewed, consciousness that resists the emasculation of self by the dominant ideology—raised consciousness—has been transformed into one that is a consciousness of active opposition—empowered consciousness.[2] For me, "empowered consciousness" means acting collectively to empower others. This may mean educating people, creating disturbances, confronting institutions, seeking group power here and there in churches, schools, communities, institutions. Empowered consciousness insists on the active, collective contestation for control over the necessities of life: housing, school, personal and family relationships, respect, independence, and so on.

Persons with empowered consciousness may still see only part of the larger world but understand they can and should influence it. This does not mean that they want to be leaders. It does mean that they want to empower others. These people see the connections between themselves and others and begin to recognize a level of universality that was obscured in their consciousness. They begin to speak of "we" instead of "I" or "they." Some of these activists are motivated by personal experience (poverty, harassment, institutionalization, a personal loss, rape, indignity, etc.). Others are motivated by something they have learned in school or out of an outraged sense of social injustice that has been fostered, for example, by families or religious beliefs. Most people are politically active for a combination of these and other reasons. A consciousness of empowerment is growing among people with disabilities. It is, in Cheryl Marie Wade's words, being passed around on notes, and it has to do with being proud of self and having a culture that fortifies and spreads that feeling:

Disability culture. Say, what? Aren't disabled people just isolated victims of nature or circumstance? Yes and no. True, we are far too often isolated. Locked away in the pits, closets, and institutions of enlightened societies everywhere. But there is a growing consciousness among us. . . . Because there is always an underground. Notes get passed among survivors. And the notes we are passing these days say, "There's power in difference. Power. Pass the word." Culture. It's about passing the word. And disability culture is passing the word that there's a new definition of disability and it includes power. (1994:15)

In *The Making of the English Working Class*, E. P. Thompson showed how workers, extraordinarily exploited and oppressed, became empowered through a culture that reflected their everyday life. This learning took place in coffee shops, bookshops, taverns, and churches. A radical culture evolved out of destitution and illiteracy. People collectively bought newspapers that were read aloud in taverns, they held discussion groups about topics of interest, and they wrote and sang songs about their lives. Thompson sums up by noting, "Thus working people formed a picture of the organization of society, out of their own experience and with the help of their hard won and erratic education, which was above all a political picture. They learned to see their lives as part of a general history of conflict" (1963:712, 795n). Self-help groups and webs of affiliation, the passing of notes and development of a history, the creation of alternative images and language, the contestation of reactionary systems—all contribute to the evolution of a necessarily resistant counterculture. A liberatory culture, in fact, that is both the reflection and the reinforcement of empowered consciousness.

Although many groups with minority or borderland experiences have created alternatives by developing cogent expositions of their own history and culture, this has not been the case for people with disabilities. This has begun to change. It is now possible to see a similar formation of "a picture of the organization of society" for people with disabilities. Carol Gill in her article "Questioning Continuum" wants to construct such an alternative picture:

In sum, I believe disability is a marginalized status that society assigns to people who are different enough from majority cultural standards to be judged abnormal or defective in mind or body. . . . But in the ideal world, my differences, though noted, would not be devalued. Nor would I. Society would accept my experience as "disability culture," which would, in turn, be accepted as part of "human diversity." There would be respectful curiosity about what I have learned from my differences that I could teach society. In such a world, no one would mind being called Disabled. (1994:44–45)

The barriers to progress are considerable and complicated. The weight of history is burdensome. The outcome is not certain. Over time progress will be made. The growing number of disability activists throughout the world testifies to that (see chapter 8). Any significant increase in the degree of consciousness and control people with disabilities experience is rooted in the mobilization of grassroots disability activism through a common language, common experiences of oppression, a developing culture and identity, and the contact with and organic formation of liberatory ideas and politics. Nancy Hartsock's prescription for changing the relationships between power and knowledge is just as applicable to the DRM as it is to the activists that she addresses: "The critical steps are, first using what we know about our lives as a basis for critique of the dominant culture and, second, creating alternatives. When the various 'minority' experiences have been described and when the significance of these experiences as a ground for critique of the dominant institutions and ideologies of society is better recognized, we will have at least the tools to begin to construct an account of the world sensitive to the realities of race and gender as well as class" (1990:172).

The Politics and Philosophy of Empowerment

The politics and philosophy of the disability rights movement have evolved out of an emerging consciousness of political activists worldwide. They incorporate the interconnected principles of empowerment and human rights, integration and independence, self-help and self-determination. The meaning of these concepts and where they programmatically lead can, not surprising, be different and, more noticeably, have different strategic importance. This reflects the divergent and often conflictual politics of the movement's activists.

It has only been in the last ten years that these political differences have affected the strategic thrust of the movement because it is only recently that a critical mass of activists, taking up a wide array of disability-related issues, has existed. The nature of the DRM's direction is at stake. For while the DRM continues to grow, it is still small and its "Let's all get together" ideological center of gravity is soft and shallow. The experience of the U.S. DRM is instructive because it encompasses the politics of different groups and leaders who have many years of practice to compare. They are, in the order of their size and influence,

- activists who have a *liberal political orientation* and relate to issues through some disability-related organization or professionals in related fields such as social services, academia, or government who have disabilities or are parents of disabled children;

- activists who have a *moderate or conservative political orientation* and relate to issues through the above channels;

- militants who have confrontational, nonideological (Alinsky-like) politics and are mainly active on specific issues like members of ADAPT (see chapter 8);

- leftists who may be involved with ADAPT, academic/policy study, or independent living centers;

- rich people (with disabilities) or people connected through philanthropy.

In the beginning the politics and organization of groups within the DRM, especially the philosophy and development of centers for independent living, were a radical break from traditional agencies. A radical philosophy of empowerment drew activists or people who wanted to be activists into the CIL networks and other groups within the DRM. Today this is not as much the case. Most CILs do not hire politically active people, do not have organizers, and have no strategic view of how to effect social change. Many executive directors of CILs and disability rights groups are apolitical, outside narrowly defined disability-related issues. Most disability rights groups avoid demonstrations because they are considered outdated or because they would alienate funding sources. A notable example of this was the pathetic response of a coalition of Michigan centers for independent living to the 1995 ADAPT demonstrations in East Lansing, Michigan's capital city. The statewide organization not only did not support the militant demonstrators in demanding increased personal assistance funding and the reform of the nursing home industry, they condemned the actions in a letter to the governor. In general, along with the rest of society, the DRM has experienced a general rightward slide. The questions about how the principles of empowerment and human rights, independence and integration, and self-help and self-determination are practiced in the evolving life of the DRM will be influenced by these political considerations.

Empowerment and Human Rights

Empowerment, of course, implies power, some kind of power. Empowerment must translate into a process of creating or acquiring power. When power is taken, it is taken from someone. Some-one loses. Within the U.S. disability rights movement, many leaders pro-mote the idea that people with disabilities can gain power without caus-ing others to suffer a loss. This leads many activists to conclude that those opposed to disability rights are mistaken or uneducated. Other "minor-ity" movements have learned firsthand that significant progress engen-ders reaction from the dominant culture. This backlash has everything to do with winning and losing. In the United States, women and African-Americans have experienced such a backlash throughout the 1980s and 1990s. Affirmative action, education, business set-asides, and multicul-tural "correctness," however marginal, have cut into the privileges that white men enjoyed for centuries. There is little doubt that white men have lost as women, African-Americans, and others have gained.

A similarly mistaken view about power and winning and losing is the notion, thoughtlessly recited within the DRM, that disability rights will not be expensive for businesses. Indeed, the Americans with Disabilities Act (ADA) was sold to the politicians on the basis that accommodations needed by people with disabilities would cost very little (a strategy I had no problem with). This flies in the face of reality. If all entities in the United States came into compliance with the ADA, it would cost a great deal. The reason laws protecting people with disabilities, like laws pro-tecting workers and the environment, are not complied with is that the interests of the bottom line run counter to them. Instead of backpedal-ing on the question of costs, a few activists forthrightly argue that they do not care how much it costs to comply with the ADA because civil rights should be guaranteed.

Empowerment, for most people in the DRM, means that people with disabilities should have more options and equality of opportunity. The latter is a favorite slogan of Disabled Peoples' International. Unfortu-nately, it is an empty slogan because it fails to take into account the dra-matic differences in opportunity among people without disabilities. The slogan fails to recognize privilege. The most extreme example is a com-ment made by Koesbiono Sarmanhadi, a leader of DPI-Indonesia, in an interview in Jakarta: "I come from a military family. I have gone to good schools in Indonesia and Australia. I know the art of politics, but when I was proposed for the national assembly, I was turned down because I am blind." The discrimination Sarmanhadi experienced in being denied a titular post in a neofascist government should elicit little sympathy.

The issue of human rights is possibly the best example of the ambi-guity of empowerment. "Human rights" implies economic, political, and social standards that insist on a minimally acceptable quality of life. Linking the issue of human rights to disability has real potential because it raises three crucial and interrelated issues: (1) democracy—are people included in decision making? (2) equality—is the distribution of wealth fair? and (3) sovereignty—is the international distribution of power uneven? Local and national elites do not want to consider the issue of democracy. They want to control who is included in all decision making. Transnational firms do not want to address the issue of equality. They are making super-profits and do not want anybody raising questions about the increasing poverty and pauperization of the world's people. U.S. political elites who control the world's dominant military power do not want to address the issue of sovereignty. They want everybody to believe that the "age of imperialism" vanished with Vietnam. Each of these issues raises questions about the systemic relation of power to oppression. Each heralds the need for resistance to the status quo. But the influence of liberal orthodoxy on the DRM and its ideological embrace of that status quo (the capitalist world order) is a real harness on its ability to take up human rights as a primary demand. It would call into question activists' own privileges, patriotism, and prejudices.

Human rights raises thorny questions: Do people have a right to sovereignty without foreign intervention? Is the right to work a basic human right?[3] The fundamental issue of human rights, a demand the DRM often makes but can never fully pursue, foretells the approaching impasse of the DRM: the DRM in the periphery can only stress human rights on an international level because it wishes to steer clear of its own, antidemocratic political elites; the DRM in the center, particularly in the United States, stresses civil rights, which steer clear of the hegemonic role of transnational capital and U.S. imperialism. Both are dead ends.

Independence and Integration

From its beginnings, the DRM championed independence and integration as cornerstones of its political philosophy. In 1983, the (U.S.) National Council on the Handicapped (NCH), in its annual report, *National Policy for Persons with Disabilities*, defined independence as "control over one's life based on the choice of acceptable options that minimize reliance on others in making decisions and in performing everyday activities" (NCH 1983:3). Furthermore, the desire of people with disabilities to take control of their lives and live in the community is conditioned by empowerment. The National Council on Independent Living (NCIL), later in 1983, published another statement on independence for disabled people: "The obstacles to a disabled person's independence can, for the sake of simplicity, be placed into three broad categories: The physical . . . ; the internal [self-esteem]; and the external [human and civil rights]. The fundamental basis for independence, indeed, its essence, lies in the latter two categories and together, they form the concept of empowerment" (NCIL 1983). The views of the NCH and NCIL are characteristic of that period and are still influential among activists. As we can see, independence was closely associated with consciousness (self-esteem) and civil rights (integration). Integration had been the goal of the civil rights movement in the United States for thirty years. It imagined the transformation of racist America into a color-blind, difference-free world. This perspective has had a lasting influence on the U.S. DRM.

Although it was probably clear a long time ago that the goal of full integration of African-Americans or people with disabilities was not achievable, the principle of integration continues to be worthwhile for the DRM. Efforts in its pursuit have produced a series of important and dramatic advances for people with disabilities in the United States in the form of policy, legislative, and legal initiatives encouraging integration in public transportation, public education, and public access (communication, architectural, commerce). Some of these measures also extended civil rights protection to people with disabilities. These activities peaked in the United States with the signing of the Americans with Disabilities Act in 1992. Many countries in Europe, notably England, continue to push for similar legislation. History will judge the effectiveness and efficacy of these initiatives.

During the same period, the organization and programs promoting independence and integration meant something slightly different to activists in the Third World. Both had more to do with political independence and economic survival because the political and economic realities were different. Whereas in the United States and Europe independence and integration were constrained by limited options and segregation, in the periphery these same goals were addressed in a void of options and intense social isolation. The struggle to realize the tenets of independence and integration can reveal the way in which politics and philosophy are differentiated by politics and place. How students with disabilities are educated is one example.

Most disability-related demands involve equal access to education. That is, the DRM demands students with disabilities be educated in "regular" classrooms. More radical activists go farther, arguing that the entire educational system is a mess and a reflection of the overall values and priorities of the dominant culture—that inclusion and integration are just parts of a necessary restructuring of public education that must occur. Of course, the integration of education, while a limited vision, would represent significant progress.

In the Third World, activists must fight to get students with disabilities educated in whatever setting will take them. This involves arranging for students to be carried up steps, using other students as readers or interpreters, or even advocating for a student to go to a segregated classroom. While the DRM supports integration, activists in many places often must settle for something much less.

Political differences within the DRM are complicated but not irreconcilable. Public transportation may be the best example of the effective collaboration of various elements in the United States. In the early 1980s disability rights activists through American Disabled for Accessible Public Transit (ADAPT) and other local groups began demonstrating against city and regional public transportation agencies and their national trade organization, the American Public Transit Association. Others, from the conservative Paralyzed Veterans of America to progressive public interest lawyers such as Tim Cook in Philadelphia, filed lawsuits charging discrimination on the basis of "separate, not equal." In addition, policy advocates began formulating local, state, and federal legislation mandating accessibility features for public buses. One by one, the collective pressure bore fruit, and city transportation agencies began to make concessions.

Again, the realities of underdevelopment require a different approach. Putting lifts on main-line buses, except possibly in more developed mid-sized cities, is not a viable solution. The number of people requiring public transportation is too large and the majority of transportation options offered to the public are privatized. The *tuk-tuks* of Asia and the *peseros* of Mexico will never be accessible.[4] The practical question, what will work and how it will bring more independence for people with disabilities, is constantly before the international DRM.

Finally, it should be pointed out that the pivotal position of independence and integration has been challenged by some within the DRM. In "Discrimination on the Basis of Disability," four well-known scholars on disability maintain that the political goals of the DRM have tended to ignore individuals' particular needs by promoting our "sameness" at the expense of our real differences (Tucker 1994). They argue that the DRM's civil rights agenda is passé because all that can be accomplished through this agenda has been accomplished. They want the thrust of the DRM to now center on the prideful and redeeming aspects of people's differences based on their disability. Unfortunately, the proponents of a "third wave" movement incorrectly conclude that much has been accomplished by the DRM's "second wave" civil rights politics. They confuse the idealist goal with the powerful principle of integration. The fact is that the advances of the DRM in the arena of civil rights must be consolidated or they will be plowed under by the inevitable politics of backlash. The logic of a third wave politics mirrors the argument made by Iris Young in *Justice and the Politics of Difference*: "Today in our society a few vestiges of prejudice and discrimination remain, but we are working on them, and have nearly realized the dream those Enlightenment fathers dared to propound" (1990:157). The idea that only vestiges of prejudice remain is not only wrong, it is misleading.

Times change, and the reassessment of political principles is vital for growth of any movement. But integration and independence must continue to be linked to empowerment. The Chicago psychologist Carol Gill and the British singer Johnny Crescendo have reframed these powerful political principles more constructively than the more trendy politics of difference. Gill: "The struggle shouldn't be for integration, but for power. Once we have power, we can integrate whenever we want." Crescendo: "We're looking for interdependence, not independence. We're looking for power, not integration. If we have power, we can integrate with who we want" (Brown 1995:150).

Self-Help and Self-Determination

Self-help and self-determination are the most radical of disability rights political principles. They are the principles that the existing power structure is least able to accommodate. Fortunately, they are cornerstones of disability rights in both the center and the periphery. These political principles are what has given the DRM its liberatory character. They separate old ideas about disability from new ideas.

The call for empowerment is ambiguous. The demand for civil rights can be accommodated through unenforced legal mandates. Few openly oppose integration. It is not always easy to draw lines of demarcation on these principles. Self-help and self-determination, in contrast, are simple and clear-cut. They require people with disabilities to control all aspects of their collective experience. They simply mean: we are able to take responsibility for our own lives, and we do not need or want you to manage our affairs; we best understand what is best for us; we demand control of our own organizations and programs and influence over the government funding, public policy, and economic enterprises that directly affect us. The demand for self-determination provocatively and intuitively attacks the ideology of paternalism; the existing political elite and power structure; social institutions like family, school, the medical establishment, social agencies, and charities; and the political, economic, and social dependency people have been forced into.

Self-help has been a crucial movement principle for twenty years. It recognizes not only the innate ability of people with disabilities to control their lives but also the innate inability of able-bodied people, regardless of fancy credentials and awards, to understand the disability experience. Self-help means everything from one-on-one peer counseling, rap groups, and independent living skills training to economic development projects like supermarkets and industrial production, collective gardening, and commercial ventures. It usually encompasses the former in the United States and Europe and the latter in the Third World. These differences appropriately reflect the different political-economic realities in the world.

These principles are not without risk. They tend to promote a go-it-alone approach that would require people to actually take control of their lives, an endeavor for which many people with disabilities are not prepared. Analogies of failed efforts at deinstitutionalization of people with mental illness come to mind. As a practical matter, self-help and self-determination are illusory short-term goals but extremely important and powerful demands.

Conclusion: A Turning Point

All the organizations within the DRM have a few basic things in common. Most important, they are organizations controlled by people with disabilities. They each, in their own way and in their own circumstances, are confronting the everyday realities of disability oppression. Another crucial similarity is that each embraces the general philosophical principle that people with disabilities must have their own voice and have control in their lives.

The politics and organization of disability rights is bound up in the dialectic of oppression and empowerment. The phenomenal growth of these organizations is unprecedented. It can be explained by the logic of oppression and its counterpart, resistance. For the first time in the history of people with disabilities, massive poverty, self-alienation, isolation, discrimination, and desperation are being challenged by the liberatory politics of the disability rights movement.

The history of people with disabilities has reached a turning point. This watershed is the result of efforts of people with disabilities, without and in spite of others. Out of their own oppression, by learning from other oppressed people's struggles, and by taking part in struggle themselves, activists in the DRM have begun to tear down an entire ideological system based in paternalism and medicalization. To date, however, there is no clear understanding of the basis of that ideological system. In the end, the only successful way to tear down an ideological system is to systematically attack its political, economic, and sociocultural foundation. Identifying and strategically chipping away at this foundation is a critical challenge for the DRM, for it threatens to undermine the energy, moral authority, and unity of the DRM itself. The forces of oppression are strong and far exceed the present strength and capacity of the international disability rights movement. Nevertheless, activists will continue to struggle for a better world. There is no alternative. The question that remains unanswered is, how successfully?

CHAPTER 8

The Organization of Empowerment

Out of the different and often hard realities of everyday life, organizations of people with disabilities have appeared in virtually every country in the world. Most of these organizations embrace the principles of empowerment and human rights, independence and integration, and self-help and self-determination, and these organizations form the core of the international disability rights movement. This development parallels, although to a much lesser degree, the process of consciousness and organization that gave rise to many kinds of liberation movements. As Sheila Rowbotham reminds us in *Women's Consciousness, Man's World*, "The vast mass of human beings have always been mainly invisible to themselves while a tiny minority have exhausted themselves in the isolation of their own reflections. Every mass political movement of the oppressed necessarily brings its own vision of itself into light" (1973:27).

In a few places people with disabilities have been politically active for many decades, but in most the disability rights movement is a recent phenomenon. Today, most activists locate the beginning of what constitutes the contemporary disability rights movement in the early 1970s.

Two years are milestones, 1973 and 1981. It was during the early seventies that people with disabilities in the United States and Europe, influenced by and directly involved in antiwar, student, and civil rights movements, began to organize on disability-related issues. Many activists, especially in Europe, Africa, and Latin America, were also influenced by leftist politics. Throughout southern Africa, where the DRM began on that continent, the influence of national liberation movements was important. Many of these people began to make political connections between their own lives and other social conditions and events.

Rachel Hurst: "Vic Finklestein is a really interesting man from South Africa who had joined the Communist party there. After he sustained a spinal cord injury, and after he had been in prison for some time, he escaped and moved to England. He was one of the founders of the Union of Physically Impaired Against Segregation in 1975. He was one of the first people to understand our segregation because he had seen segregation so starkly in South Africa. We owe him a great debt."

Ed Roberts: "So much of the good that has happened to me and the good I've done has to do with being in Berkeley in the sixties. There was such energy, so much optimism. We were the generation that could and would change the world. There were all sorts of alternative living experiments and new ideas. Like everybody else, I just got caught up in them. Fortunately, there were other people with disabilities who were also affected. We were together at the right time at the right place."

The period from 1972 to 1973 is associated with the founding of the Berkeley Center for Independent Living. It was also about then that the Boston Self-Help Center became interested in independent living as an alternative kind of organization. The independent living movement has been the linchpin of the DRM in the United States, and its leaders have had an influence on activists and leaders elsewhere. The first rights-oriented group in Europe was established in England when Vic Finklestein, Paul Hunt, and others initiated the Union of Physically Impaired Against Segregation in 1975.

As activists in the United States and Europe began to take up major disability-related issues, the DRM began to develop and grow. Early on these issues included the inaccessibility of public transportation; the lack of accessible, affordable housing; the institutionalizing of poor, young people with severe disabilities in nursing homes because of the prohibitive cost of personal assistance; the struggle for inclusion of students with disabilities in regular classrooms; and efforts to change the way in which the public relates to, perceives, and understands disability. The last area is pivotal because it calls into question the dominant mythology about disability.

Although the first center for independent living began in Berkeley in 1973, most CILs in the United States were set up in the early 1980s.

There are now more than three hundred. CILs are the most important organizations within the U.S. DRM for two reasons. First, most of the early disability rights leaders were identified with CILs, and the philosophy of independent living formed much of the basic philosophical underpinnings of the larger DRM. Second, CILs were and still are cornerstones of the DRM because of the sheer numbers of paid staff. These centers have extensive resources.

Out of the work of early activists, legislation and legal mandates concerning the "handicapped" appeared. This happened in North America and northern Europe and to a lesser extent in the Third World. The most important in North America was the Rehabilitation Act of 1973.[1]

The year 1981 was designated the International Year of Disabled Persons (IYDP) by the UN. The significance of this was lost on most disability rights activists in the United States. While I do not know if this was the case elsewhere in the center (I doubt it), 1981 was very important to the DRM in the periphery. In many cases, it was the first time efforts were made to involve people with disabilities in disability-related projects and programs.

Narong Patibatsarakich: "In 1981, the International Year of Disabled Persons, Thailand had its first workshops about disability that people with disabilities actually participated in. At the end of that year, I was selected to go to Singapore for the Disabled Peoples' International Congress. Before this meeting, I had no ideas about philosophy, politics, and so on. . . . When I heard Ed Roberts speak, he had a big impact on my ideas. When I came back to Thailand I was committed to starting DPI-Thailand. First, we meet with alumni of the deaf schools to get them organized. Next, we met with the Parents Association of the Mentally Retarded. Then I started the Association of the Physically Handicapped. One year later, we met and formed DPI-Thailand. We had our first Congress in Chiang Mai in 1983."

In Third World countries where disability-rights organizations were established prior to 1981, the IYDP provided a certain momentum. In summarizing a history of disability rights in Brazil, Eugene Williams writes, "As a consequence, in 1980 Brazil hosted the first National Meeting of Entities of the Disabled with nearly one thousand participants representing the blind, deaf, [physically] disabled and Hansen diseased. Guidelines for action were established and also the foundation of a national coalition in an attempt to encompass the areas of disability. Moreover, a new policy was defined for the following year, the IYDP. The policy consisted of representation by disabled people and not by the 'specialists'" (1989).

Indeed, a crucial event had taken place earlier than the IYDP in late June 1980 when there was a split in Rehabilitation International, the most significant disability-related international body. RI is a large membership organization composed primarily of rehabilitation professionals. Through efforts of people from Sweden and Canada, RI, for the first time, made an attempt to bring people with disabilities to its conference in Singapore. The largely token effort backfired. The few hundred participants who had disabilities demanded that RI mandate that 50 percent of its Delegate Assembly be composed of people with disabilities. This motion was overwhelmingly defeated by a vote of 61 to 37, a vote that probably represented the sentiments of the three thousand other delegates at the convention. Those with disabilities and a few supporters led a split in RI, the outcome of which was the formation of Disabled Peoples' International.[2] DPI has seen impressive growth in the last fifteen years. There are affiliated groups in dozens of countries and an international headquarters in Winnipeg, Canada.[3] Joshua Malinga, who later became DPI's general secretary, and Danilo Delfin, who later became a paid organizer for DPI, attended the Singapore conference as observers from Zimbabwe and the Philippines, respectively. Their experience is representative of many who attended.

Joshua Malinga: "When I went to Singapore I was conservative, but when I returned I was very radical."

Danilo Delfin: "The Singapore conference had a big impact on me. I realized I wasn't so disabled, that it was possible to have a family and work. After that conference I started working on disability issues full time."

The conference had an electric effect on its disabled participants. DPI was propelled by this initial stimulus and its message of community control and self-representation: "The prerequisite for successful action lay in the proper organization of a disabled persons group, and the development of a high level of public awareness of disability issues. . . . [O]ur organization should assert that they were the true and valid voice of disabled people and our needs" (DPI 1986).

Although progress is uneven, it is undeniable. Within the last fifteen years, self-help groups have formed in leprosy communities in southern Africa, in refugee camps in Kampuchea and Mexico, and on remote islands in the Philippines, Palau, and Fiji. A village in the mountains of Mexico is controlled by people disabled from drug-related violence, and has attracted hundreds of people with disabilities from throughout the country. Economic development projects like supermarkets and agricultural collectives have been set up in Africa by these organizations. The first centers for independent living have appeared in a number of cities in South America. Most of these groups are relatively new, small, and fragile. Their roots are in the 1980s. Most exist without funding or developed programs. Others, like the National Council of Disabled Persons Zimbabwe and Disabled People South Africa, are quite sophisticated organizationally and politically.

Most of the organizations of the DRM were founded between 1979 and 1986. The National Council of Disabled Persons Zimbabwe, initially registered as a welfare organization, became a national disability rights group in 1981; the Organization of the Revolutionary Disabled was set up in the wake of the Sandinista victory in 1979; the Self Help Association of Paraplegics (Soweto) (SHAP) was started in 1981 as an economic development project; the Program of Rehabilitation Organized by Disabled Youth of Western Mexico (PROJIMO) also began in 1981 as a rural community-based rehabilitation (CBR) program; DPI-Thailand was established in 1983; the Southern Africa Federation of the Disabled (SAFOD) was formed in 1986 as a federation of non-governmental organizations of disabled persons; and so on. It was during this time that most centers for independent living, as well as many other disability rights groups, including ADAPT, were established in the United States.

The experience in Brazil is typical:

Towards the end of the 60's and into the 70's disabled persons began to take the initiative and formed athletic and social clubs such as the Clube do Otimismo (Rio), Clube dos Paraplegicos (Rio and São Paulo), SADEF (Rio), and ARPA (Rio Grande do Sul) that were, and are today, characterized by revenue-producing activities such as silk-screening, sales of lottery tickets and selling candies in the streets and by highly competitive wheelchair basketball teams. While these groups were not overtly political in nature, they were important focal points for discussion, socialization and building a sense of community and met other needs. . . . During the eighties the self-help movement surpassed national borders and had the Organização Nacional de Entidadas de Deficientes Fisicos (ONEDEF) represent Brazil at Disabled Peoples' International, by way of its Latin American Council. The blind became affiliated to the World Blind Union (WBU) and to the Latin American Blind Union (LABU). Similarly, the deaf, through FENE-SIS, are now part of the World Federation of Deaf, expanding their political influence and improving their leadership. . . . 1984 was a crucial year for structuring the organization. A series of entities were founded: Brazilian

Federation of Entities of the Blind (FEBEC); National Organization of Entities of People with Physical Limitations (ONEDEF); National Federation of Education and Integration of the Deaf (FENESIS); and the Reintegration Action Group of Hansen Diseased (MORHAN). Additionally, a Brazilian Council of Entities of People with Disability was founded in December of that same year to lump the four entities. New associations 'of' people with disability began sprouting all over the country. (Williams 1989)

From many disparate beginnings and places, networks began to form. They were established in Brazil in the 1980s and later throughout South America. Conferences have been held in Rio de Janeiro incorporating individuals and organizations throughout the continent. There are national coalitions in South Africa, Zimbabwe, India, Thailand, and numerous other countries. Members of DPI-Thailand and DPI's regional organizer, Danilo Delfin, based in Bangkok, have made numerous trips to Vietnam, Laos, and Kampuchea to spread the philosophy of disability rights and to initiate activities. There have been international exchanges between Hong Kong and the People's Republic of China.

Over the years, organizational progress has been uneven. As we have witnessed much progress, there have also been setbacks:

Following the celebration of the International Year of Disabled Persons in 1981, the Government of the Philippines through the then National Council Concerning the Welfare of Disabled Persons, convened in 1983 the first National Congress of Disabled Persons. . . . [T]he Congress established the first national organization. . . . However it did not succeed fully for the following reasons: (a) the members of the governing board were based mostly in Manila; (b) the organization had no support framework, i.e., funds, office, communication facilities and staff; (c) unity among members of various disability groups could not be achieved and factionalism and conflict of interests prevailed. (Estrella 1992)

As Danilo Delfin told me, "Keeping the momentum of 1981 has been very hard."

Disability rights activists have made different choices over the years on how and what to organize. In 1991 people with disabilities in Rio de Janeiro set up the first center for independent living in South America. This was followed by another CIL in São Paulo, with the likelihood of others forming throughout South America. In South Africa the Federation of the Deaf produced the first sign language manual in Africa and has been sending people to the United States and England to learn sign language. In Bombay, the India Federation of the Blind has a huge modern taping and braille facility. The National Council of Disabled Persons Zimbabwe has established economic development projects like a supermarket in a township outside Bulawayo and collective gardens outside Harare. DPI-Thailand staged demonstrations criticizing the Thai government for dismissing a deputy cabinet member who used a wheelchair. One of the first things the Organization of Disabled Revolutionaries (ORD) did after the Nicaraguan revolution was to set up a wheelchair production and distribution system using locally available materials in their wheelchair design.[4]

Many of these organizations started as a response to the simple need for survival, and their goals were limited to economic self-help and self-sufficiency. Others started as political groups that wished to mobilize people with disabilities in their communities, cities, countries, or regions. These groups and purposes have gradually merged. All seek to link their work with the struggle for self-determination and human rights. With few exceptions, this is their common denominator.

A Typology of Disability Rights

As people with disabilities began to organize, they worked on priority issues that were considered feasible. More often than not, the organizations have grown or died as a result of these decisions. Reviewing the various structures and strategies organizations of the DRM have adopted delineates the following typology: (1) local self-help groups (LSHGs), (2) local advocacy and program centers (LAPCs), (3) local single issue advocacy groups (LSIAGs), (4) public policy groups (PPGs), (5) single issue national advocacy groups (SINAGs), (6) national membership organizations (NMOs), (7) national coalitions/federations of groups (NC/FGs), (8) national single disability organizations (NSDOs), (9) regional organizations (ROs), and (10) international organizations (IOs).

LOCAL SELF-HELP GROUPS

LSHGs vary from small collectives of people providing peer counseling and moral support to small plot gardening and agricultural ventures to larger projects involving a significant level of support, production, and revenue. Many LSHGs do not have a developed disability rights agenda. They may be concerned only about their members. Many activists consider LSHGs outside the DRM, but most of these groups have helped a lot of desperately poor people with severe disabilities and often they are affiliated with larger disability-related organizations. Some, like the Program of Rehabilitation Organized by Disabled Youth of Western Mexico, have served as a model for other self-help groups. PROJIMO was established in 1981 as a rural community-based rehabilitation program by the Palo Alto, California-based Hesperian Foundation. PROJIMO became very well known in Mexico during the 1980s, serving as a model for eight other CBRs in different parts of Mexico (as well as others throughout the Third World). David Werner's *Disabled Village Children,* which grew out of the PROJIMO experience, has been translated into thirteen languages and is used worldwide.

In South Africa, there are more than 175 revenue-generating self-help projects, most associated with Disabled People South Africa. Most employ less than thirty people and yield little revenue. However, the projects generate a minimal level of food or income for its members which often is the margin between life and death. The largest and best known is the Self-Help Association of Paraplegics/Soweto, established in 1981 by a group of Soweto paraplegics (primarily spinal cord injured) led by Friday Mavuso. SHAP is membership driven. The chairperson and the executive council are elected by the members at the end of each fiscal year. Members are people with disabilities in Soweto. A management committee headed by the chairperson meets monthly. SHAP is an affiliate of Disabled Persons South Africa.

Very similar to the experiences of other groups such as Mexico's PROJIMO, Nicaragua's ORD, and Rio's CIL, many of SHAP's core members met each other in the Baragwanath Hospital outside Johannesburg. Like PROJIMO, these people began to organize a self-help group out of their own desperate situations. The first project was a factory, started in 1983 in Mofolo Park, adjacent to Soweto, with funding from major South African companies and trust funds. At its height in 1989, the factory employed 140 people. Workers, in teams of eight, supervised by a person with a disability, did electrical assembly, sewing, packaging, and repair work. SHAP also had programs on housing, education, health, and recreation (including a sports club). Subsequently, SHAP organized peer counseling and sports programs (mainly racing and basketball).

The experiences and lessons from the hundreds of self-help groups are diverse. The peer relationships and friendships, material aid and support, and sense of control they engender have significantly contributed to the health and sustenance of hundreds of thousands of people. These groups are the easiest to establish but the hardest to maintain. Of the ten types of disability organizations that come under the umbrella of the DRM, LSHGs are the most transitory.

LOCAL ADVOCACY AND PROGRAM CENTERS

The most important LAPCs are centers for independent living.[5] CILs are nonresidential, not-for-profit organizations that engage in advocacy, service, and public education activities. The advocacy is both systemic and individual oriented. There are hundreds of CILs in the United States and northern Europe. In addition, a handful of centers exist in the Third World. The Centro do Vida Independente (CVI), which opened in 1990 in Rio de Janeiro, was the first CIL in the Third World. Its political roots were in earlier national advocacy groups like the Movimento Pelos Direitos das Pessoas Deficientes (Movement for the Rights of Disabled Persons). CVI provides work training, architectural and legal advice, databank services, peer counseling, therapeutic and support aids, independent living skills training, and cultural and recreational activities. They publish a newsletter *Super Ação*. In 1992 CVI began to coordinate international symposiums on disability. These "Ibero-American Meetings of People with Disability" have been attended by disability rights leaders throughout the Americas. By definition, CILs must work on behalf of all disabilities and a majority of their boards of directors must be people with disabilities.

Access Living of Metropolitan Chicago (AL), where I have worked since 1985, was founded in 1979. It is one of the largest CILs in the United States, with a budget in excess of $1.8 million and forty staff members. The organization's budget revenue comes from city, state, and federal government grants along with private sector funding from foundations and individuals. AL's president, Marca Bristo, is one of the country's best-known disability rights leaders. A former chairperson of the National Council on Independent Living, she was appointed chairperson of the National Council on Disability by President Bill Clinton in 1993.

Access Living assigns a significant number of staff solely to advocacy and organizing activities. In addition, AL provides support to the local ADAPT chapter as well as support for progressive issues such as domestic violence, housing discrimination, child abuse, and health care reform, all issues that are important to people with disabilities. The primary issues AL addresses are housing, personal assistance, public transportation, health care, and education. Consumer services are quite diverse and include information and referral (20,000 calls annually), individual and group peer counseling, independent living skills training, and individual advocacy training and support. These "core services" are provided by most CILs. AL also provides domestic violence emergency intervention, housing legal services, and various kinds of public awareness activities like lectures and media campaigns. Seventy percent of AL's 1,400 (annual) consumers are African-American, and more than 85 percent are on fixed incomes of under $10,000 a year. Although a majority have a physical disability, a significant number are deaf and mentally ill. AL is one of many LAPCs in the Chicago area working on disability rights.

LOCAL SINGLE ISSUE ADVOCACY GROUPS

Many local self-help groups appear spontaneously and as quickly disappear. The same can be said of LSIAGs. The major difference between the two groups is that LSIAGs are advocacy oriented while self-help groups are principally concerned with individuals' livelihoods. Many LSIAGs align themselves, sooner or later, with larger advocacy organizations, which helps to sustain them.

These groups concern themselves with a wide range of issues, from housing and transportation to accessibility and public awareness. Acesso Libre is an LSIAG in Mexico City. Their advocacy, as the organization's name indicates, deals with architectural accessibility. South of Mexico City in Oaxaca, the Asociación Solidaria de Personas con Limitaciones Fisicos de Oaxaca (ASOPELFI) was born out of a need to advocate for employment and wheelchairs for its members. By the time the group had expanded to sixty active members, it was dealing with many advocacy issues in the city of Oaxaca. The evolution of an LSIAG is well described by Fadila Lagadien, a founder of People with Awareness on Disability Issues (PADI) in South Africa.

Fadila Lagadien: "I met Kathy Jagoe who was a high-level quad who had moved to Capetown and had lectured about disabilities in different parts of the world. Kathy suggested that I start a disability awareness group and, with her help, we started People with Awareness on Disability Issues. This experiential workshop lasted for a couple of years, and many issues came up, like transportation and accessibility, but mostly we talked about disability awareness. We started to use computers to communicate our issues. Then we decided to start a newsletter because attitudes about disability are so bad.

I got a volunteer who was from Texas whose husband was working in Capetown to help with computerizing the newsletter. . . . So after a lot of work, we now produce a 24-page newsletter that we mail to three thousand people throughout South Africa. We have been invited to places like Zimbabwe and Canada to talk about our experiences. We have the idea to set up an independent living center now. PADI is a small organization that is an affiliate of DPSA."

PUBLIC POLICY GROUPS

There are many public policy-related centers, institutes, and projects that relate to disability. Few are controlled by people with disabilities. Most are government, quasi-government, foundation, or academic based. There are a few controlled by people with disabilities that are key components of the DRM. In the United States the Disability Rights Education and Defense Fund, based in Berkeley and Washington, D.C., played a crucial role in formulating and organizing for the landmark Americans with Disabilities Act. In Hong Kong the Joint Council on Disability Programs (JCDP) was successful in developing two policy "papers" that were the basis for Hong Kong's Rehabilitation Program Plan that included an oversight Rehabilitation Development Coordinating Committee.

The World Institute on Disability (WID), founded by Ed Roberts, Judy Heumann, Joan Leon, and Hale Zukas in San Francisco's East Bay in 1984, is an international public policy, research, and training center. The institute has developed educational and leadership training programs throughout the world from Latin America to the former USSR. Many of the institute's staff have spent considerable time outside the United States promoting disability rights. WID has convened international forums and foreign exchanges on personal assistance, leadership training, and disability rights philosophy. Their conferences on personal assistance services and technology have included disability activists from many places. They also have produced a series of important documents, books, and videos on funding PA services, the implications of emerging technologies for people with disabilities, and independent living. The organization has also become well known for its work on connecting AIDS services and advocacy into the larger disability advocacy networks.

WID is funded from government and private sources. Its office is located in Oakland and has a staff of thirty-five. Ed Roberts and Judy Heumann are among the DRM's most noted and celebrated leaders.

Many have called Roberts the "father of independent living" because he founded the first CIL in the United States, the Berkeley Center for Independent Living. Heumann has been just as important to the U.S. disability rights movement, especially in her work as a national figure in the independent living movement. In 1993 she became the Assistant Secretary for Special Education and Rehabilitation Services in the Clinton administration. Ed Roberts died in 1995, leaving serious questions about the future direction of WID.

SINGLE ISSUE NATIONAL ADVOCACY GROUPS

Although there are many local single issue advocacy groups, there are few on a national level. This is because of the difficulty of organizing people over great distances on a particular issue over time. It is expensive and hard to identify common targets. Communication and organizational democracy are difficult as well. I do not know of any SINAGs in the Third World, but this type of organization has proved important to the DRM in the United States because of the outstanding contribution made by ADAPT.

ADAPT was founded in Denver in 1978 by the late Wade Blank, a radical minister and political activist influenced by Martin Luther King, Jr. Initially, Blank had organized a group of severely disabled people, many living in nursing homes, to establish a new kind of collective community that allowed many to break out of the dependency of nursing home life. Their community was called Atlantis. The first issue Atlantis and other disability rights activists took up in Denver was making public transportation accessible. After a series of militant demonstrations, public meetings, and negotiations, ADAPT/Atlantis won. This was a turning point for the U.S. DRM because it demonstrated that a small group of activists could win major concessions regarding public services and policy.

Interest in ADAPT grew, and a national organization was founded in 1983 by activists from Denver, Chicago, Austin, Atlanta, and a few other cities. Blank and Mike Auberger became the most identified leaders of national ADAPT, which continued to be coordinated in Denver. ADAPT now has active chapters in many cities. Blank recently died, but others such as Auberger, Mike Ervin in Chicago, Bob Kafka and Stephanie Thomas in Austin, and Mark Johnson in Atlanta continue to provide a loose sense of direction to ADAPT's chapter network. ADAPT has continued its confrontational tactics.

ADAPT was probably the most important disability rights group in promoting the issue of accessible transportation efforts, which led to the accessible public transportation provisions in the ADA. Since 1992 ADAPT's focus has shifted to the general area of personal assistance services (PAS), with particular emphasis on redirecting government funding for nursing homes to home-delivered, consumer-controlled personal assistants. ADAPT also has been involved in national health care reform and its potential for funding PA services and long-term care services.

Organizationally, ADAPT operates with little formal national structure. Its ambivalent political philosophy is scattered through its newsletter, *Incitement*. Many of ADAPT's leading members are consciously left, although the group does not have a strong ideological orientation.

Many ADAPT chapters do excellent ongoing work on the local level; others are dormant until ADAPT's annual or semiannual national demonstrations. Historically, ADAPT has provided a militant pole around which activists could unite. Unfortunately, given the conservative and apathetic political environment and (to a lesser degree) the inclination of ADAPT's unofficial leadership not to lead, ADAPT has not noticeably grown in the last five years. ADAPT continues to have between three hundred and five hundred active core members, with another layer of people they influence.

NATIONAL MEMBERSHIP ORGANIZATIONS

NMOs have local chapters through which its membership participates in advocacy and program activities as well as organizational business. Most NMOs are quite democratic, although there is a strong tendency to follow the same leadership over extended periods.

Most of the organizations discussed throughout this book are NMOs: Disabled People South Africa; Asociación para los Derechos de Personas con Alteraciones Motoras (Mexico); Organización Revolucionarios Deshabilidades (Nicaragua); Asociación Cubana Limitados Motor Fisicos Nacional (Cuba); National Council of Disabled Persons Zimbabwe; Disabled Peoples' International-Thailand; and Persatuan Penyandang Cacat Indonesia (Indonesian Disabled Peoples Association). I will briefly touch on a few because of their importance.

The Organization of Disabled Revolutionaries grew out of the Sandinista revolution that came to power in Nicaragua in 1979. Many of the founding members of ORD met at hospitals and the municipal rehabilitation center in Managua. An early influence on ORD was a delegation of politically progressive people with disabilities from the San Francisco Bay Area who visited Managua in the winter of 1980–1981. Many of ORD's leaders were Sandinista (FSLN) militants who became disabled during the armed struggle against the U.S.–backed Somoza dictatorship. ORD was given a large house (abandoned by owners who fled to Miami) in the center of Managua by the FSLN government and began to develop self-help programs and do outreach. ORD's membership soon swelled to thousands of people throughout the country, with some active local groups reaching into remote rural areas. ORD received some initial funding from international foundations, principally to establish a wheelchair production and repair shop. ORD also distributes medical equipment and coordinates sports, cultural, transportation, and public education programs. During the late 1980s, ORD began to fragment. A number of other disability-related groups emerged to address particular issues. These groups—CEPRI, Pipitos, and Solidez—were formed in 1986, 1987, and 1988, respectively, to provide information on disability (CEPRI), education for Downs syndrome children (Pipitos), and employment assistance (Solidez). These groups work well together on many issues.

Disabled Peoples' International-Thailand was formed in 1983. DPI-Thailand was the second NMO in Southeast Asia to join DPI. During its first decade, DPI-Thailand's efforts concentrated on public education, leadership training, and legislative advocacy. The focus in the latter area has been on employment and architectural access. The organization also publishes a newsletter and has developed a handbook on disability rights. DPI-Thailand has a small budget and two salaried officers. The Executive Committee meets every three months to direct the staff. An annual meeting is held to elect a chair and the executive committee. Activists in DPI-Thailand regularly participate in regional DPI activities, principally the expansion of DPI-affiliated self-help groups throughout the countryside and in neighboring countries. Contacts were established in Vietnam, Kampuchea, and Laos in the early 1990s.

The Indonesia Disabled Peoples' Association (IDPA) has much in common with disability groups throughout East Asia, namely, its close association with the ruling political party. What makes IDPA particularly interesting is that the organization's structure is a mirror image of Indonesia's ruling party. That is, the association's membership chooses its chairperson through a representational congress (which meets every five years), and the chairperson appoints all officers, committees, and staff, approves all publications, and mandates and directs the organization's activities. IDPA was formed in 1987 and is an affiliate of DPI. There are twenty-seven local branches (one in each province). The chairperson/secretary general of IDPA, Otje Soedioto, has access to all of Indonesia's politicians. Soedioto, a lawyer, is a personal confidant of Indonesian dictator Suharto and represents him on particular legal matters. IDPA's orientation is strict cooperation with the Suharto regime.

The constitution of the National Council of Disabled Persons Zimbabwe's (NCDPZ) spells out the organization's mission: "[to] promote full integration into Zimbabwean society of all disabled persons and active participation by the disabled in the planning and decision-making processes that affect their own lives." NCDPZ leaders are widely recognized throughout Zimbabwe. Joshua Malinga, NCDPZ's founder, is the mayor of Bulawayo, Zimbabwe's second-largest city. Alexander Phiri and Ranga Mupindu are also nationally recognized figures.

Members meet locally on a regular basis as NCDPZ branches and elect their own leaders. Leaders and activists from the branches compete for election to the National Executive Committee of NCDPZ which consists of fifteen members. They, in turn, elect their national officeholders, set policy at the national level, and appoint an executive director. The national office is in Bulawayo and has a salaried staff of eighteen people with disabilities. The work of NCDPZ involves advocacy, grassroots organizing, services, and leadership development training. NCDPZ has been able to obtain funding from foundations located in northern Europe. These foundations support specific programs or purchases, such as personal computers or agency vans.

NATIONAL COALITIONS/FEDERATIONS OF GROUPS

As the number of DRM organizations multiplied, networks were established to unify efforts on a national basis. These national coalitions operate like federations, ensuring the autonomy and equal input of each group. For example, NCDPZ consolidated its strong links to the Zimbabwe Sports Association of the Disabled, the Zimbabwe National League of the Blind, and the Zimbabwe Down's Children's Association by initiating the Zimbabwe Federation of the Disabled (ZIFOD).

In the United States, the National Council on Independent Living (NCIL) was initiated in 1980 and formally established in 1982 to link CILs and advocate on their behalf. NCIL has a national office in

Washington, D.C., with a small staff. Its main function in the last decade has been to represent CILs in the U.S. Congress and in government funding agencies. For example, NCIL has been the crucial advocate on the questions of what criteria should define CILs, how and when CILs should be federally "accredited," how federal funding should be dispersed to CILs, and what kind of reports CILs should be required to submit to government agencies. NCIL also funds a computer information project that disseminates appropriate information through the Internet.

The British Council of Disabled Persons (BCODP) is a coalition of 110 organizations controlled by people with disabilities. The BCODP encompasses England, Wales, and Scotland. While there is uneven development between the urban and rural areas, the overall organization is quite strong. BCODP includes caucuses and groups that have specific concerns, for example, gays and lesbians. There is a regionalization program that manages from the grassroots level. BCODP is affiliated with DPI. NCIL and BCODP, like other NC/FGs, hold national meetings to choose leadership, provide information, prioritize issues and resources, and conduct its other business.

NATIONAL SINGLE DISABILITY ORGANIZATIONS

NSDOs are the oldest, most traditional type of disability organization. Most disability activists would consider most of these groups to be outside the DRM because they are not controlled by people with disabilities, they are often deferential to government or philanthropic organizations, and they tend to be apolitical. They are close to but not identical with charities. A few have made significant contributions to empowering people with disabilities, albeit with a single-disability focus. These few NSDOs actively work in coalition with other disability rights organizations and can be considered part of the DRM. One such NSDO, the National Association for the Blind–India (NAB), established in 1947, is the largest disability organization in India with seventeen state branches (out of a total of 25 states). The NAB was instrumental in setting up the National Society for Equal Opportunity for the Handicapped. The NAB plays a crucial role in the Rehabilitation Council, a federal advisory group on disability. The leaders of the NAB, such as Rajendra Vyas, are important figures in India's DRM.

The NAB's first major project was the consolidation of India's braille system. This accomplishment inspired UNESCO, under the leadership of Sir Clutha McKenzie, a New Zealander, to standardize braille worldwide.

Today, the NAB provides training in education and mobility to people in 800 to 1,000 rural villages each year. The major activities at NAB's central headquarters are policy development, networking, public education, book brailling, and audiotape reproduction. The NAB is India's most prolific producer of braille books and audiotapes. NAB reaches as many as 400,000 blind people annually.

NAB meets once every three years in a general assembly. There an executive council is elected. The executive council appoints committees for NAB's work (books, braille technology, employment, women, etc.) and also directs the program activities. According to the NAB's by-laws, at least five members of the fifty-member council must be blind. In 1993 nine of the fifteen officers were blind. State branches are divided into districts and subdivided into *tabulaks*. That year the NAB's budget was 8 million rupees, 13 percent of which came from the national government.

REGIONAL ORGANIZATIONS

ROs are also federations of groups. They function quite like NC/FGs, except they are not national in scope. Some, like the Illinois Network of Centers for Independent Living (INCIL), which links CILs in the state of Illinois, encompass small areas. Other ROs, like the regional disability coalition in Europe, the Federation International des Mutiles des Invalides du Travail et des Invalides Civils, and the Southern Africa Federation of the Disabled, are independent federations.

SAFOD represents disability rights groups in Angola, Botswana, Lesotho, Malawi, Mozambique, Namibia, South Africa, Swaziland, Zambia, and Zimbabwe. The aim of SAFOD is to provide a forum for disability rights activists to meet, share common concerns, and coordinate regional projects. According to SAFOD, activities are designed to "support the formation of disability related organizations, the training of disabled people to be leaders of these groups and to facilitate exchange of information in the field of disability through public education programs, seminars, travel and exchange, conferences, and publications concerning all aspects of the lives of disabled people" (1993).

SAFOD has a secretariat in Bulawayo, Zimbabwe, with a small staff headed by a secretary general. It has received funding mainly from northern European foundations like OXFAM. SAFOD is a member organization of Disabled Peoples' International. SAFOD is governed by an executive committee, elected at each biannual General Assembly and drawn from the national organizations.

SAFOD's Regional Development Plan for Southern Africa includes public education, self-help, accessibility advice, small-scale enterprises for economic development, training and exchanges, and a women's regional development program. It also widely circulates its newsletter, *Disability Frontline*. SAFOD has been particularly effective in establishing disability rights groups throughout the southern cone of Africa. A major outcome of these efforts was a 1991 conference in Harare, Zimbabwe, where forty delegates came from all over Africa to discuss disability issues. The crucial achievement of the meeting was the adoption of the "Harare Declaration on the Establishment of the Pan African Federation of Disabled People," signed by all the attending delegates. The SAFOD manual, *Development Activists Handbook* (by Machenzie Mbewe and Peter Lee), has been used throughout the region as an important leadership training guide.

INTERNATIONAL ORGANIZATIONS

There are a growing number of disability rights organizations that do international work. Some, like Mobility International, based in Eugene, Oregon, provide opportunities for activists with disabilities to visit other countries. These exchanges have been very successful in spreading the experiences of independent living, peer counseling, and self-help projects and an awareness of the politics of disability across many cultures. Another important international organization is Action on Disability and Development (ADD), based in London. ADD has established contacts in 152 countries, 121 of which are in underdeveloped countries. Seventy-eight percent of all ADD's newsletter readers contact them at some point, demonstrating that people are desperate for information, peer contact, and support.

There has been a great deal written here about Disabled Peoples' International, the most important IO, so I will only briefly add to these comments. DPI was founded in Singapore in 1981. DPI's programs emphasize leadership development, community organizing, and self-help. Through its leadership, most prominently chairperson Henry Enns, DPI was involved in the formulation of the UN's *World Program of Action Concerning Disabled Persons* in 1982 as well as the UN's Decade of Disabled Persons (1992–1993). More than seventy countries have DPI chapters. The membership of DPI consists of national assemblies. Any national organization that is controlled by disabled people can be a member of the national assembly of that country.

Participation of individual countries in world affairs is through a regional structure. DPI member countries are divided into five regions: Asia/Pacific, Africa, Europe, Latin America, and North America/Caribbean. Each regional assembly meets at least every two years and elects five persons to the World Council. The World Council has the responsibility for all activities undertaken by DPI.

The Disability Rights Movement as a Counterhegemonic Popular Social Movement

Where does the disability rights movement fit within the politics of social change? Is it important or irrelevant? Is it liberatory and transformational or limited to its own parochial issues? Does it have a subversive character, and if so, what can it subvert? Are there lessons other political activists can learn from the politics and organization of the DRM? There are more questions than answers, and some of the answers, at least those answers that I can suggest, are partial and not necessarily encouraging.

One way to assess the DRM is to identify the social milieu in which it commonly operates and then compare it with other movements operating in a similar milieu. This domain is most commonly thought of as civil society. Today, we are witnessing an explosion of books, movies, and discussion about civil society. At the center of civil society are what some have come to call "intermediate institutions." These institutions are nongovernmental, often voluntary bodies and include schools, community organizations, charities, and church groups. Some people have argued that these institutions are the greatest promoters of democracy and that people should become involved in them. Some estimate that 89 million adults in the United States give an average of four or more hours per week to these institutions (*Nation,* February 26, 1996, 15).

Parallel to this phenomenon is the emergence of what have been called "popular social movements" (PSMs). These movements are focused on a set of issues that have to do with controlling immediately necessary resources, including housing, land, food, the environment, and the body. PSMs range from very large movements for women's rights, civil rights, and environmental protection to midsize movements of landless peasants or literacy campaigns to smaller organizing projects of block clubs, cab drivers, and student associations.[6] A major question is whether these new political formations will achieve an influence that will enable them to reach their objectives and have the staying power to maintain them.

Only recently have political activists begun to understand that political power must be contested on the levels in which intermediate institutions exist. Control over these institutions may hold one of the keys for relatively marginalized forces to begin to transform their lives. This recognition is an important political contribution made by popular social movements. Immanuel Wallerstein summarizes this point in *Transforming the Revolution*: "Once we recognize that in practice power is enormously diffuse, we can see the conquest of power by the family of antisystemic movements involves far more than the conquest of state power, which if not secondary in importance, may at least be secondary in temporal sequence. Whatever strategy we construct must give up this blind faith that controlling the state apparatus is the key to everything else; it may well be that everything else is the key to controlling the state apparatus" (Amin et al. 1990:47).

In arguing that the disability rights movement is a popular social movement, two British disability rights scholars, Mike Oliver and Gerry Zarb, use Carl Boggs's summary of the critical traits of PSMs that mirror those of the DRM: "To varying degrees and in varying ways the new movements also seek to connect the personal (or cultural) and political realms, or at least they raise psychological issues that were often submerged or ignored" (Boggs 1986:51). Oliver and Zarb go so far as to make the assertion, "Hence, the disability movement will come to have a central role in counter-hegemonic politics and the social transformation upon which this will eventually be based" (Oliver and Zarb 1989:237). Although I question the contention that the DRM will have a central role in counterhegemonic politics, I believe that the emerging politics and organization of disability empowerment leaves little doubt that the DRM is a popular social movement, and an important one at that.

What makes the DRM subversive is paradoxically the extraordinary worldwide oppression of people with disabilities. The oppression is systematic. The principles, demands, and goals of the DRM cannot be accommodated by the present world system. These aspirations, when fully considered, lay bare the concealed horror of that world system and dominant culture. Although the DRM cannot subvert that domination in its totality, it can and does chip away at it, in the immediate institutions of everyday life. Time will tell if the powerful principles and convictions of the DRM will help to produce a long-term transformation of that domination.

PART IV

Conclusion

Many who readily accept my conclusion that racism is here to stay are unsure what they should do with this unhappy knowledge. "If racism is permanent," they ask, "then isn't struggle hopeless?" The answer is as difficult as the question. Struggle to gain full acceptance in this country, for all black people—as opposed to some black individuals—is virtually impossible in a society as we know it. But the obligation to try and improve the lot of blacks and other victims of injustice (including whites) does not end because final victory over racism is unlikely, even impossible. The essence of life fulfilled—a succession of actions undertaken in righteous causes—is a victory in itself.

Derrick Bell, *Faces at the Bottom of the Well*

CHAPTER 9

The Dialectics of Oppression and Empowerment

Chronicling the theory and practice of any liberation movement tempts a prejudgment of that movement's ultimate success. Derrick Bell's assertion of the permanence of racism impressed on me that such claims are often erroneous, even disingenuous. Regrettably, as the permanence of racism appears probable to this legal scholar and political activist, so does the permanence of disability oppression to me. I do not draw this conclusion indifferently. People with disabilities have much experience with different social systems and cultures and a preponderance of signs point to this conclusion. This is not, as many have accused Derrick Bell, a defeatist existentialism. It is, I believe, a reasonable and pragmatic appraisal of the expanse and depth of disability oppression in its political, economic, cultural, and psychological manifestations.

There are, nevertheless, two sides to the "permanence" of disability oppression. On one side is the capacity of oppressive structures and institutions to reproduce themselves through the myriad power relationships in everyday life. On the other side is the inevitability that oppression will generate its opposites—resistance, empowerment, and, from these, potentially, liberation and freedom.

It is not easy to think about social phenomena in terms of dualities or paradoxes and contradictions, but reality is complex and contradictory, no matter how much we yearn for something simpler. Dialectics is a way of thinking that comprehends this incomprehensibility, that penetrates paradox, and resolves or at least accommodates contradiction.

Although our everyday lives show us how these contradictions are played out—love and hate, happiness and sadness, rich and poor, victory and defeat; the dominant culture tries, with alarming success, to "teach" us something different. We are taught to think in terms of isolated incidents and fragmented facts that stand still in time. The possibilities that a defeated strike can lead to greater political victories (for example, the outbreak of a successful revolution) or that a wheelchair, a symbol of dependency, can be the provider of great independence are ludicrous following the logic of the dominant culture.

Dialectics is predicated on something we know intuitively, that everything in life—politics, economics, art and culture, our individual beliefs and our very psyches—is constantly in flux. Dialectics is the best method for understanding oppression because its essence is change and oppression is a changing condition. The opposition to oppression is also a process, a process of recognition, identity, education, and resistance. If we were to take an optimistic but also realistic perspective, we might summarize the dialectic of disability oppression as follows: within the impossibility of the real end to disability oppression lies the possibility, even the probability, of significant political and social progress. It is in this context that I conclude by elaborating on (1) oppression in relationship to empowerment, the challenge to build a movement that unites as many people as possible; and (2) oppression in its relationship to liberation and freedom, the ultimate goals of such a movement.

Oppression and Empowerment

A fundamental paradox confronting the disability rights movement is that the progress of people with disabilities is contingent on significant economic development (the accumulation and expansion of capital) and, correspondingly, the emergence of (more) modern ideas about disability (the influence of capital) and, at the same time, the development of a movement that insists on social justice and equality (the restriction of capital) and an epistemological break with the dominant ideology (the rejection of capital).

Oppression is experienced both individually and collectively. No one person experiences a unique kind of oppression. This is because oppression is a social phenomenon and all social phenomena are either structured or influenced by political-economic and sociocultural factors. It is this dualism—individuality and collectivity—that is at the heart of personal and social transformation. People's struggle against oppression unites them in the most material and spiritual ways. This struggle *incorporates their differences,* but, paradoxically, it also *differentiates them.* During the course of empowerment two things are going on: individuals are changing, and society is changing. Individuals necessarily, regardless of volition, begin a personal search for self-identity whenever they fight back, whenever they work to change their world.

It is on these dual levels that the accommodation (maybe not full resolution) of the contradictions between the individual and the collective, difference and unity, the personal and the political, is found. The internal struggle of a movement to achieve the broadest possible unity while supporting its activists' individual quest for self-identity must become motive forces in any liberatory effort or project. This contradiction between individual and collective goals must be accommodated or that movement will fail. This, unfortunately, has not been done with much success so far in other liberation movements. This contradiction is not irreconcilable. Whether we talk of struggle for a better life on a personal level or on a social level, these struggles are intrinsically political. This is one of the great lessons of the feminist movement: the personal is political, and the political must be personal.

This lesson can be extended to help resolve the contradiction between the individual and the collective, a relationship that is, at once, the basis of all liberation movements and one of their most difficult challenges. The question of how individuals long isolated by political, economic, and social marginalization can find one another and unite around their common experiences of oppression while accommodating one another's profound differences has an often perplexing history. The contradiction between the individual and the collective is particularly complex among people with disabilities because of our isolation, stigmatization, and fragmentation into categories (MS, MD, MR, MI, ED, EMH, LD, CP, SCI, deaf, late-deaf, hard-of-hearing, blind, visually-impaired, and so on).

There is a wide spectrum of experiences among people with disabilities that are filtered by class, gender, and race. Because disability oppression, like all human experience, is experienced between real people and not between people as individuals and structures as collectivities, social transformation requires that there must be a collective change in the way individuals think and behave.

The individual's relation to the collectivity is not a new subject. Jean-Paul Sartre's critique of Marxist orthodoxy in *Search for a Method* was published in 1968. Sartre sought to rescue Marxism from its one-sided fixation on the collective when he wrote, "It is precisely this expulsion of people, their exclusion from Marxist knowledge, which resulted in the renaissance of existentialist thought. . . . Marxism will degenerate into a non-human anthropology if it does not reintegrate people into itself as its foundation. . . . From the day that Marxist thought will have taken on the human dimension (that is, the existential project) as the foundation of anthropological knowledge, existentialism will no longer have any reason for being" (1968:179, 181).

Sartre's efforts were successful. The radicalism of the late sixties, not only in France but around the world, resonated with an interest in human and personal development, creativity, and responsibility. These movements did, albeit unevenly, maintain a coherent direction and have a great deal of success in forcing the dominant culture into structural and ideological changes. Sartre's insistence on the individual was not meant to undervalue the collectivity. He never pitted them against each other but always situated them in relation to each other. Undoubtedly, there is a phenomenology of oppression—a phenomenology that exists at both the individual and the collective levels.

In chapter 6, I suggested that the failure of most people with disabilities to identify with other people with disabilities is the principal contradiction that limits the DRM's potential influence and power. The relationship between the commonalities and differences in the disability experience goes to the heart of the identification question, raising fundamental issues for the DRM.

The notion of difference within disability is almost always missing in the major research on disability. This is the case in Erving Goffman's influential book *Stigma*. Goffman not only depoliticized the oppression of people with disabilities, he treated disability as uniform. Goffman's deviance theory failed to comprehend the divergent forms and experiences of oppression because it did not recognize differences among people with disabilities. One only has to ask simple questions to raise serious doubts about its explanatory power. For example, what about those with hidden disabilities (is cancer "stigmatized" only if people gossip?), or the "stigma" status of a destitute, black, gay man with AIDS? Does deviance theory help us to understand why a nonverbal Mexican immigrant with cerebral palsy dies mysteriously in a Chicago hospital after an alleged experimental treatment? Why do Maoris with renal failure find no access to dialysis? What about the class, race, or gender differences within disability? Does anyone imagine that a black sixteen-year-old boy with a spinal cord injury received from a gunshot, who lives in a housing project in Brooklyn, experiences the same stigma or stereo-type "problems" of a sixteen-year-old spinal cord-injured white girl who was hurt in a diving accident and lives on Martha's Vineyard?

As Adrienne Asch and Michelle Fine noted in their introduction to *Women with Disabilities,* "To date almost all research on disabled men and women seems simply to assume the irrelevance of gender, race, eth-nicity, sexual orientation, or social status. Having a disability presumably eclipses these dimensions of social experience. Even sensitive students of disability (for example, . . . Goffman 1963) have focused on disabil-ity as a unitary concept and have taken it to be not merely the 'master' status but apparently the exclusive status for disabled people" (1988:3).

The problems with theories that disregard differences within social groups are primarily twofold. First, such theories situate oppression in the knowing subject: one can be oppressed only if one knows one is op-pressed. This implies that membership in an oppressed group is limited only to those who identify with that group. You cannot experience the stigma of disability unless you think of yourself as having a disability. You do not experience stigmatization unless you "feel" it. For the DRM, this distinguishing criterion is important. Second, if this kind of identity theory is correct, oppressed groups are reduced to clusters of interested individuals who can only be interested in their own needs. The DRM in this sense becomes an "interest group," like unions, pro-choice groups, tobacco growers, and thousands of other groups interested in a partic-ular policy, budget, or law. We are not oppressed; we have neglected needs. Again, these efforts emasculate the essence of disability oppres-sion. They place disability in the "needy" category (those who need) as compared to a "have" category (those who have). People are not op-pressed. They are stigmatized by an uneducated public and therein have unmet needs.

Recently we have witnessed the opposite error. Instead of framing the question of oppression only in terms of the collectivity of a particular group, which obliterated the profound differences within that group, all sorts of books and articles have appeared which frame the question of oppression only in terms of the individual. This postmodern or poststruc-turalist position revels in diversity. By seeing difference everywhere, its ad-herents must reject unifying commonalities anywhere, except at the most discrete levels. In the end, society is just too complex, human experience too singular to allow any (meta)theory of disability oppression.[1] When universality is abandoned, when difference becomes everything at the expense of collectivity, only the lonely, isolated individual remains. This perspective, like the one it is so determined to repudiate, continues to pit the individual against the collective and refuses to appreciate the dialectical relationship between them.[2]

In his article on postmodernism and Marxism, Manning Marable, a leading African-American social critic, charts a third course, "transformation." Marable distinguishes two historical tendencies within the African-American community: inclusion (associated with civil rights advocates Frederick Douglas, Martin Luther King, Jr., and Roy Wilkens); and black nationalism (associated with Marcus Garvey, the young Malcolm X, and Huey P. Newton). Marable's alternative paradigm, transformation, is associated with W. E. B. DuBois, Paul Robeson, Fannie Lou Hamer, and the older Malcolm X. Marable writes that transformationists

have sought to deconstruct or destroy the ideological foundations, social categories, and institutional power of race. Transformationists have sought neither incorporation or assimilation into the white mainstream, nor the static isolation of racial separation, but the restructuring of power relations and authority between groups and classes in such a manner as to make race potentially irrelevant as a social force.... This critical approach to social change begins with a radical understanding of culture.... Culture is both the result and consequence of struggle; it is dynamic and ever changing, yet structured around collective memories and tradition.... To transform race in U.S. life demands a dialectical approach toward culture which must simultaneously preserve and destroy. We must create the conditions for a vital and creative black cultural identity in the arts and literature, and in music and film.... But we must also destroy and uproot the language and logic of inferiority and racial inequality. (1995:86)

This third paradigm has much to offer people with disabilities and the disability rights movement. It locates ideology (of inferiority, false consciousness, and the failure of identity) on a systemic level—in oppression. It also argues for the possibility of an organized resistance to people's common oppression—empowerment. Transformation offers the real possibility of resolving the contradictions between the individual and the collective constructively. Only by simultaneously constructing our own identity as people with disabilities and destroying the categories that separate and differentiate us as a group can we transform our own collective realities as poor, powerless, and degraded individuals.

Oppression and Freedom

What is the strategic goal of the disability rights movement? Is it strictly human rights, or is it liberation and freedom? What exactly would liberation be like for people with disabilities? What is the best way to go about ending disability oppression, and on what basis do we struggle for social change? Is the demand *Nothing About Us Without Us* a genuine, liberatory call for self-determination or a plea for recognition by the dominant culture? What are the barriers to liberation and freedom, and what are the challenges for the disability rights movement? Do the necessities of everyday life provide the resources and practical experience to fashion a more liberatory existence, or do they act as fetters to progress? There are many questions with many answers.

Freedom seems to be the only true negation of oppression. It is a condition free of oppression. For some, freedom is an absolute condition. For others, freedom is not an absolute state or a state of mind. It is predicated on an evolving recognition by people of what they need and how to satisfy those needs. As Friedrich Engels wrote in *Anti Duhring,* "Freedom is the recognition of necessity" ([1878]1972:167).[3] This is a real-world proposition not separated from a state of mind but bound up with it. Liberation and freedom must be understood as processes, for they transform the individual and collectives' material and spiritual necessity.

Need is not a desire or a want. It is a socially ordered (configured) condition. For example, personal hygiene is a universally valued need. This need can be easily met for those with modern bathrooms. But consider the hundreds of millions of people who do not have modern bathrooms. In many cases, simple necessity is not so simple.

A more vital need is drinking water. Every tourist who visits the Third World is told not to drink the water. In Mexico, the result of failure to comply is called "Montezuma's revenge." In fact, you cannot drink the water because of the social priorities of the elites. It is not because Third World countries do not have sanitary engineers. It is because it is too costly for the elites, and besides they can make a lot of money on bottled water. You can bet the water that comes out of their taps is as good as any in the United States or Europe. The point is that the social conditions of, in this case, underdevelopment prevent tap water from being pure. Of course, poor people drink the water, so it is not surprising that the diseases associated with drinking contaminated water (hepatitis A, cholera, parasitic infections) are prevalent throughout the Third World.

In many of these countries, parasitic infections are not even treated. Because they are seen as a chronic medical condition, they are not treated, for the medical procedure is considered a waste of time.

The necessity of water acquisition is not just a sanitary problem. In Soweto, a visitor immediately notices women and children with buckets lined up at the water spigots. Many of the houses do not have running water, so there are water spigots every four or six blocks. Necessity is not an individual thing, it is socially conditioned. In a conversation I had with Albie Sachs, an executive committee member of the African National Congress (ANC) and now a member of South Africa's Supreme Court, he mentioned that although when the ANC took power, the transition to redistribute resources would be done gradually, immediate efforts would go into increasing public water spigots to make water gathering easier.

Further, necessity is not a progression of needs like housing, safety, good health, friendship, family, community, and respect. Nor is it a hierarchy of needs or simply survival. It is a complex social whole, ordered and determined by the whole itself, by life's social conditions, by society. Society governs necessity. A necessity to people in one place (like a fireplace) might be considered a luxury to others; a luxury in one place (like a telephone) might be considered a necessity somewhere else. To recognize necessity requires an understanding of society, but to understand society you must engage it, act on it, change it, and at some point have some control of it. Most people do not have enough control of their lives. Without control, people cannot master necessity or at least key aspects of it.

It is readily apparent that the elites, as individuals and as a class, recognize their necessity and act on it. This may mean military intervention, trade or currency agreements, propping up foreign dictators with "aid," crushing strikes or settling them, repealing or even enacting progressive legislation. It may mean increasing wages or cutting them, increasing interest rates or cutting them. The list is long. They have a lot of "freedom" and they know it is linked to power and control and they are constantly fortifying it. They know their necessity (power, freedom) is bound up with the whole of society. An inevitably changing society requires them, as individuals and as a class, to influence or direct that change as much as possible. They are not apathetic or apolitical.

Most people do not recognize the conditions of their necessity. It is opaque in the sense that they see it but it is blurred. They know from experience how to survive and also recognize many of the elements necessary for them to get beyond subsistence. The capacity to challenge the crushing limits or borders of their lives appears beyond their reach. This obscured outlook is mediated by necessity itself. People who are constantly confronted by the question of survival have little time to waste on "foolish" activity. This is a paradox that prevents people from demanding and developing greater control of and in their lives.

We can say this is generally true for people with disabilities. Their lives are extraordinarily difficult. They do not have what most of us take for granted as the most necessary elements of an acceptable life. In tandem with this condition, there is the absence of control people *feel* in their lives: a spiritual and emotional vacuum. The lack of material and emotional security creates dependency. Over time, dependence emasculates people's self-image, creativity, and productive capacity. In the (practical) activities of everyday life, dependency contradicts freedom. It can be considered the alienation of a freedom that should naturally flow from the political and personal control people have over the simple necessities of everyday life—what Sartre saw as the alienation of the potential for empowered consciousness: "In his progress from 'consciousness' to 'praxis,' Sartre has encountered necessity. This necessity, in the form of the alienation of *praxis,* can only be transcended by a praxis that is recovered in the midst of necessity" (Girardin 1972:320). The struggles of the DRM for freedom and liberation must be recognized and understood in a context bounded by the necessities of everyday life—housing, education, transportation, access, recreation, family and friendships, work, sex, and so on.

By doing so, the processes of liberation and freedom can be understood as functions of gaining greater control because, although different, liberation and freedom are bound together by necessity, by social reality. As Sartre discovered, these processes must be "engaged" by praxis. Praxis could be another term for political activism generally, or, more precisely, empowerment. Necessity creates the boundaries of the possible. Empowerment/praxis explores those boundaries, ultimately broadening them.

Freedom is also not a unidimensional condition or stage beyond necessity only truly attainable in a postscarcity society. There are degrees of freedom just as there are degrees of power and degrees of control. Each of these is fashioned in the course of everyday life and in the course of political struggle. In short, by people, in their individual and collective practices of controlling their lives. This is empowerment, or perhaps what Sartre meant by recovering praxis in the midst of necessity.

I believe the disability rights movement is a liberation movement because it has always situated self-control and community control at the center of its agenda. The history of the DRM has been the growing consciousness and activism of greater numbers of people with disabilities. Unlike many, if not all, of the progressive mass movements today, the DRM is expanding. For the first time in history, millions of people with disabilities have seen or heard about other people with disabilities who are fighting back, struggling for a better life, trying to change the wretched necessity of their existence. This is a liberatory beacon of hope for many. The praxis of empowerment means and has meant creating or increasing the options available to people with disabilities in their everyday lives. Each of the crucial tenets of the DRM—empowerment, independence, and self-help—requires considerable control. The demand "Nothing About Us Without Us" must mean something more than a petition for community input, it must be a demand for self-determination.

Freedom is not an absolute state any more than liberation is simply an event. Liberation and freedom are emancipatory processes that reach such a degree of fruition and maturity they become a generalized social phenomenon. They do not preclude individuals, even many individuals, from "advancing" (whatever this might mean) beyond or within the condition(s) of oppression prior to the maturation of a generalized social condition. A person can declare "I am free, I am liberated" and may be reasonably accurate. Liberation can be, on the micro level, experienced individually. It is also a directed process with a strategic end, Bell's "final victory." This end may come for people with disabilities, but it will come long after we are all gone. Until then, as Fanon tells us in *The Wretched of the Earth*, "to live means to keep on existing. Every day is a victory, . . . a victory felt as a triumph of life" (Murphy 1987:137).

Personal Anecdotes on the Future and the Past

I am constantly reminded that all progress is stamped with the imprint of the past. When I see old people using "walkers" I am always struck by the generation and development gaps in how people with disabilities live. Some day people will be liberated enough to discard such ridiculously antiquated aids. The idea that slowly hobbling around is better than briskly moving about in an electric wheelchair would be shocking if I did not see it practiced every day.

The other day I heard a local television news reporter say that a man had died in a fire because his wheelchair had trapped him inside. The idea that a wheelchair, a mobility aid, would trap anybody in a burning building would be preposterous to me if I did not hear the term "wheelchair-bound" every day. What seems to me the most elementary evidence of oppression, that a fellow wheelchair user died because he lived in an inaccessible building and was always, every day, trapped by this condition, resonates with clarity.

Whenever I travel to the Third World, I am asked by other people who use wheelchairs about the light manual chair I use. If they have financial resources, they ask me where they can get one. If not, they ask if there is a way one could be donated.

It is my belief that a traveler can gauge the level of economic development and the level of organization among people with disabilities based on what kind of wheelchairs they see being used. The lack of modern, appropriate wheelchairs seems to me a blatant violation of human rights, similar to the lack of housing and food.

Today, people with disabilities are categorized from the onset of their disability. All of a sudden we are less. In chapter 1 I referred to this as "shrinking." This is the way Susan Sontag described it and probably felt it when she was diagnosed with cancer. This is how Rachel Hurst described it the very moment she went out into the world using a wheelchair. This is why Nancy Ward of Nebraska People First says people should never be labeled because it automatically puts limits on them. Some day all the labels (ED, LD, EMH, DD, MR, MI, etc.) and all the programs (special education, special services, Special Olympics, etc., etc.) associated with these labels will be tossed in history's dustbin.

We disability rights activists know all these categories are phony. We have felt what Pierre Bourdieu calls "the real function of classification systems" (Dirks, Eley, and Ortner 1994:155).[4] They oppress the people they define. They do so on two levels. First, they imply we are inferior. Second, they allow the dominant culture to institutionalize those of us they consider outcasts and misfits. The best example of this is the classification and "treatment" of mental illness. Taxonomies of this kind have been used by all power structures we know of—from those associated with slavery and mid-nineteenth-century capitalism to the twentieth-century Soviet institutionalization of antistate noncoformists (Gamwell and Tomes 1995, esp. p. 105).

Whenever I consider the raised consciousness of my friends and comrades with disabilities, I know we, a relative few, have been liberated from a terrible weight of history. Strangely, we are living with the ideas of the future. I am constantly reminded of just how close we are to so many others, just like us, forcibly, oppressively locked in the past. The future never arrives, but the past can be slowly extinguished. The old, antiquated ideas and categories will some day vanish.

Challenges and Choices

On one level, this book is about challenges and choices, or more precisely, the abundance of challenges and the scarcity of choices. The dilemma most people with disabilities throughout the world face is how to use their meager resources to attend to this condition. So the most obvious challenge is the most elementary: how people with disabilities secure the basic needs to survive. For the vast majority of the 375 million people with disabilities living in the Third World this can be a matter of life and death. For those of us living in the "developed world," achieving a level of self-sufficiency goes directly to the question of quality of life.

This is not unlike most everyone else. The phenomenon of disability oppression has many similarities with class, gender, and race oppression. The paternalism of patriarchy and slave ideology are simply two striking examples of how the ideological roots of disability oppression share the same terrain that literally billions of other people have traversed. That the vast majority of people with disabilities are extremely poor, with little if any political power, also unifies our experiences with billions of others.

There is no doubt that people with disabilities experience oppression differently based on historical, cultural, and sociological factors. We have been identified, defined, and set apart by the dominant culture based on particular physical, sensory, and/or mental conditions. Because of this exclusion, these conditions are disadvantages experienced in everyday life. Furthermore, our differences often set us apart from others for one unique reason: our physical, communicative, and attitudinal environments are hostile to us. Hence our necessity also includes mobility devices and medical supplies; architectural and communication access; personal assistants, interpreters, and mobility trainers; and a different awareness about disability.

Historically, the only choice people with disabilities had in their personal struggle to survive was to individually resist isolation, even death, by relying on others. This meant, practically speaking, begging and becoming dependents of family or charities. That has begun to change. Now there is a movement of empowered people that seeks control of these necessities for themselves and their community. But this movement faces enormous challenges and choices as well. How these challenges are confronted will inform the effectiveness of the movement itself and its impact on the everyday lives of people with disabilities. These choices have life and death consequences.

In the course of grappling with an array of complex and burdensome issues, the fundamental challenge is how the movement develops politically. What kind of analysis and political program will its leaders and activists bring to their struggle? How well does the DRM link its theory and practice? How will people with disabilities become politicized? And how will the people who come forward as activists become integrated into the political work and life of the movement?

In turn, another set of strategic choices are raised. These have to do with how the disability rights movement understands and affects the political process and confronts the question of power. For systemic problems, systemic solutions must be found. This is a complicated issue. On the one hand, to believe the global oppression and pauperization of billions of people does not have a direct relationship with the state of the human condition, a condition involving 500 million people with disabilities and a condition dominated by the political economy of international capitalism, is a political dead end. On the other hand, for the DRM to grow and politically prosper, it must unite all who can be united on the principles of empowerment and self-determination. The DRM must have a broad constituency. It cannot become doctrinaire or sectarian.

All liberation movements must come to terms with these strategic choices. There is, inauspiciously, no certainty on these questions. Whereas the DRM is politically united on the progressive principles of empowerment and self-help, there is no proof that a broader political vision is evolving. A vision that helps present and future activists understand why and who they are fighting. This strategic question must be answered adequately or the movement will degenerate. It is also a question that must constantly be reexamined as the objective and subjective conditions facing people with disabilities change. The DRM has, so far, not split over questions of philosophy and power, but the potential is there. For if the DRM does not fully grasp the implications of being a liberation movement, the movement will lose its moral authority.

These challenges are made ever more difficult by three facts: the poverty and isolation of most people with disabilities; the dominant culture's capacity to project images, influence ideas, and produce consent; and the failure of alternative systems, most prominently real existing socialism, to make much of a difference in the way people with disabilities have lived. Fortunately, we can say with as much certitude that however difficult the challenges and choices are, the personal lives of disability rights activists explode the mythology of people with disabilities as passive nonpersons and confirm for us that people do and can make their own history and that the struggle of survival is a triumph of life.

Disability as Part of the Human Condition

Two children are born in New York City. A white baby boy and a black baby girl. The parents of the boy are college teachers. The baby girl is the child of a single mother on welfare. The babies have unusually similar physical characteristics, except for one. The white baby is born with muscular dystrophy. The doctor tells the black mother: "You have a beautiful baby girl." She tells the white couple: "I'm so sorry, you're baby is severely handicapped." The doctor is an African-American woman. She personally has experienced the racism and sexism that black girls and women face. She knows statistically that life for this baby girl will be full of hardship and adversity. Yet she feels greater sorrow for a white baby who will grow up in a middle-class family, get a good education, probably go to college, probably get a decent job, and probably have a better quality of life. So it goes. This example is meant to convey how deep but also how contrived and false the ideology of inferiority/superiority is.

I am constantly asked, after I have argued that disability is simply part of the human condition and intrinsically no better or worse than other aspects of that condition, if we shouldn't work to prevent disability. The expected coup de grâce is usually, shouldn't we do everything we can to prevent the birth of babies with disabilities? I answer quite seriously that this is an abstract question to me. What preconceptions do we start with, I ask in return? What particular social conditions will these particular kids grow up in? Then I pose a question in return. If we can prove statistically, I ask, that most baby girls born in certain districts of New York, Los Angeles, or Chicago or in any number of places throughout the Third World will have difficult lives, do we then start trying to prevent baby girls from being born? Of course not. We work to change the social reality those children live in. The fact that most children with disabilities face difficult lives has much more to do with the social environments they live in than their intrinsic physical or mental qualities. So the question of prevention always remains a question abstracted out of real life.

Having a disability is *essentially* neither a good thing nor a bad thing. It just is. This intrinsic "neutrality" of disability is the primary aspect of all the contradictions bound up in the condition of disability. There is, however, a secondary aspect of disability—its bad side. Disability often brings physical pain and atrophy; psychological and cognitive disorientation; inconvenience, immobility, and an assortment of other nuisances like catheters and ventilators. While this secondary aspect of disability should not be discounted, it is the perverse inversion of these aspects that essentializes disability as intrinsically inferior/bad which the DRM has attacked. By minimizing, patronizing (hero worship), and often eradicating the essential neutrality of disability, the dominant culture trivializes the intrinsic complexity of disability (just like it does everything else). Some people with disabilities want to be "cured"; others don't. Both positions can be understood as rational only if this complexity is acknowledged. The expansion of people's choices within this problematic is something, I believe, that should be considered progress.

In the real world, some people with disabilities have a generally good life and others a generally bad life. The condition of disability is a fork in the road of life with all its new and often difficult choices and challenges—not unlike the junctures that everyone else encounters. Some of the people with disabilities living a good life do so in spite of their disabilities; others may be living a good life because of their disabilities. This is the positive aspect of those that preach a politics of difference: everyone is different.

The differences are real; the categories and preconceptions are false. Although there are numerous natural differences among those with disabilities, it is on the basis of these false categories and preconceptions that the common experience of disability oppression is experienced. This paradox or contradiction—out of difference comes unity—is the basis of the disability rights movement. A contradiction that any vibrant and counterhegemonic movement must contend with and resolve in the course of its practical work.

Life itself is a series of struggles—some won, some lost. Resistance for most people with disabilities is a necessity for survival. The DRM should never lose sight of this. Throughout the course of this project, I have been impressed with how many of the stories and experiences of politically active people with disabilities reflect this proposition. We have begun to speak for ourselves, to make demands, to organize, and to educate others. And, no matter how much the dominant culture conditions us otherwise, as Alice Walker, we have begun to come to peace with ourselves:

It is thirty years since the "accident." A beautiful journalist comes to visit and to interview me. She is going to write a story for her magazine that focuses on my latest book. "Decide how you want to look on the cover," she says. "Glamorous or whatever." Never mind "glamorous," it is whatever that I hear. . . . At night in bed with my lover I think up reasons why I should not appear on the cover of the magazine. "My meanest critics will say I've sold out," I say. "My family will now realize I write scandalous books." "But what is the real reason you don't want to do this?" he asks. "Because in all probability," I say in a rush, "my eye won't be straight." "It will be straight enough," he says. Then, "Besides, I thought you'd made your peace with that." And I suddenly remember that I have.(1983:390–391)

Notes

Chapter 2: The Dimensions of Disability Oppression: An Overview

1. Einar Helander, at a press conference on the release of the United Nations Report *Human Rights and Disabled Persons* (*Chicago Tribune*, December 5, 1993). Helander has written a number of reports for the UN, including *Prejudice and Dignity* and, with Padmani Mendis, Gunnel Nelson, and Ann Goerdt, *Training the Disabled in the Community*.

2. For example, unpaid domestic labor contributes to the socially necessary sustenance and nurturance of paid nondomestic labor, and the people, prominently women, involved in this work should be considered part of the laboring class. See Ferguson 1989.

3. O'Connor does not mean to imply that people defined as surplus are unnecessary. He means they are irrelevant to the present political-economic system. The notion of surplus people was explicitly developed to account for the treatment of people with mental retardation in Farber 1968.

4. To a great extent, exiles have avoided this "declassing." They have, at least in many cases, become incorporated into new economic milieus subsequent to their forced expulsion from their homeland.

5. Much has been written about precapitalist economic formations. There have been a number of efforts to refine the classification of their primitive, feudal, or semifeudal characteristics: "archaic" (Polanyi 1944); "tributary" (Amin 1990); "precapitalist" (Dobb 1946). Many have simply used the term "traditional."

6. This is in sharp distinction not only to psychology, as discussed earlier, but also to the German idealist philosophy of Kant, Hegel, and Schopenhauer. For these people separated society and being from consciousness and thought. For example, in *The Phenomenology of Mind* Hegel extinguishes any social relationship to truth or any civil or state (government) relationship to justice. Later,

in *The Science of Logic,* he merged the two. Thought *is* being, and there is a distinction between reality and actuality.

7. Overdetermination is a theory associated primarily with Louis Althusser. Trying to avoid orthodox Marxism's theory that economic relations determine all social relations, he conceived the notion that the "superstructures" (language, law, custom, religion, etc.) have their own "specific effectivity." But Althusser argues that these distinct realities are subject to the "determination in the last instance by the [economic] mode of production," although there is "the relative autonomy of the superstructures and their specific effectivity" (1964:111). This is overdetermination. While I do not subscribe to Althusser's idea that superstructures are distinct realities (his structuralism), I do believe that overdetermination is an insightful way of thinking about relationships. In this case, while powers have their own specific effectivity, they are ordered by class rule. Once the ensemble of power relationships is configured or ordered, these relationships evolve primarily from their internal dynamics.

8. The theory of hegemony is one of the great contributions of the Italian communist Antonio Gramsci, who insisted that the principal way power was projected by the capitalist ruling class (Italy in the 1920s) was through hegemony or ideological domination. In his *The Two Revolutions* Carl Boggs argues that Gramsci's theory of hegemony penetrated the realm of power where ideology (most notably culture) and political economy met: "For Gramsci ideas, beliefs, cultural preferences, and even myths and superstitions possessed a certain material reality of their own since, in their power to inspire people towards action, they interact with economic conditions, which otherwise would be nothing more than empty abstractions" (1984:158).

9. See Paulo Freire's "banking theory" in *The Pedagogy of the Oppressed* (1973).

10. Freire is probably the best-known theorist of hegemonic practices of schooling. He has been influential in developing counterhegemonic education. He is associated with literacy campaigns in Cuba, Guinea-Bissau, Nicaragua, and Brazil. In *Ideology, Culture, and the Process of Schooling,* the critical theorist and educator Henry Giroux writes, "According to Freire, it is the cultural institutions of the dominant elite that play a major role in inculcating the oppressed with myths and beliefs that later become anchored in their psyches and character structure. To the degree that repressive institutions are successful in universalizing the belief system of the oppressor class, people will consent to their own exploitation and powerlessness" (1988:134).

Samuel Bowles and Herbert Gintis (1976), Michael Apple (1979), Henry Giroux (1988), Paulo Freire (1968, 1973, 1987), and Michel Foucault (1980) successfully demonstrate the role of schooling in the production of a monoculture and the reproduction of existing power relations. It is ironic that while the literature theorizing the hegemonic practices of schooling has burgeoned in recent years, the voices of radical educators, especially those critical theorists who have promoted such views, have been silent on disability, inclusion, and special education, where the oppression and control of students has been the greatest. While this omission of radical pedagogy does not compare to the common outrageous treatment of students with disabilities, it is just as telling of the status of students with disabilities.

11. Joseph Tropea's article, "Bureaucratic Order and Special Children," is useful because of its focus on the historical socioeconomic necessities that framed early attempts to warehouse "incorrigible, backward and otherwise defective pupils" (1987:32).

12. The same regulations that are being used to provide students with access are also being implemented in such a way that many students are being inappropriately removed from regular education, resulting in questionable educational benefit and possible harm (Gartner and Lipsky 1987). This is particularly true in the area of high-incidence mild disabilities, the so-called educable mentally handicapped, learning disabled, and behaviorally/emotionally disordered. Special education is increasingly used to segregate students labeled "mildly handicapped"—students whom schools have difficulty serving or whom they choose not to serve. These programs often have a disproportionate enrollment of racial minority students. For instance, though African-American students make up 16 percent of the public school population, they represent 35 percent of those labeled educable mentally handicapped.

13. An unpublished paper that Gill and Voss developed at the Chicago Institute of Disability Research: "Inclusion Beyond the Classroom: Asking Persons with Disabilities About Education."

14. In 1993 the magazine *Vanity Fair* ran a series on telethons. Most of the commentary centered on the "worth" of a life with disability. This brought Paul Longmore's work to the fore. Longmore, a leading disability rights academic then at Stanford University, had decisively shown elsewhere that telethons promoting charities are the principal ideological mediums transmitting and inculcating attitudes about disability in the United States. Longmore writes that the four major telethons—Easter Seals, Arthritis Foundation, United Cerebral Palsy, and Muscular Dystrophy Association—reach a combined audience of 250 million people and their message "is hegemonic in creating attitudes and ideas about disability" (Longmore, quoted in Bennets 1993:92).

15. For the purposes of this book, I use the term "language" as it is commonly understood. I recognize that Ferdinand de Saussure in his *Course in General Linguistics* distinguished "language" from "speech" to argue that language is unable to be transformed, that it is an unconscious code. Émile Durkheim argued that this "split" was the basis of society. In this sense I am most often exploring speech, although I make the point numerous times that language, as it is used, is interiorized and its meaning inculcated.

16. Some people argue that ideology is partisan in that it is inherently at the service of the dominant culture; others argue that it is neutral and a contested terrain of ideas. Just before he died, Sartre defined ideology in the former terms: "Ideology . . . is an ensemble of ideas which underlies alienated acts and reflects them. . . . Ideologies represent powers and are active. Philosophies are formed in opposition to ideologies, although they reflect them to a certain extent while at the same time criticizing them and going beyond them" (Schilpp 1991: 20). Sartre sees ideology as always partisan. Slavoj Zizek, editor of *Mapping*

Ideology, thinks ideology is more limited and more neutral: "Ideology either exerts an influence that is crucial but constrained to some narrow social stratum, or its role in social reproduction is marginal" (1994:14). For the purposes of this book it is most useful to think of ideology as a system of ideas and beliefs that are projected.

Chapter 3:   Political Economy and the World System

1. This study, *Human Rights and Disabled Persons,* commissioned by the United Nations and released in December 1993, estimates there are 290 million people with moderate to severe mental or physical disabilities in the world, 200 million of whom live in "developing" countries. This number is expected to double over the next thirty-five years, a rate that exceeds population growth because of a rising proportion of older people. The report documents that in several countries children and adolescents with disabilities are often killed or die from neglect.

2. In Southeast Asia, 80 percent of the jobs exist in five metropolitan centers—Jakarta, Singapore, Kuala Lumpur, Bangkok, and Manila. There is a great concentration of political, economic, social, and cultural capital in these cities as well. Mexico City's metropolitan area of 20 million people dominates the political, economic, social, and cultural life of Mexico. The same is true for São Paulo and Rio, Lima, Buenos Aires, Bombay, Delhi, and Calcutta, Bangkok, Jakarta, Beijing, Hong Kong, and Shanghai for their respective countries.

3. For example, the richest 20 percent of Mexicans earn fourteen times the income of the poorest 20 percent. Brazil's richest 20 percent earn twenty-five times the income of the poorest 20 percent (in the U.S., the figure is "only" 11 times). Land distribution is also illustrative. In Brazil, the wealthiest 0.9 percent of landholders own 44 percent of the land while the poorest 53 percent hold just 2.7 percent (NACLA 1995:16).

4. For example, the countries of Latin America and the Caribbean owed in excess of $521 billion by the end of 1994. See *Notimex* (July 13, 1995) and *Latin America News Update* (September 1995).

5. The Claymore is one of the most common land mines (along with two Russian models). It is made by Morton Thiokol in Shreveport, Louisiana, and sells for $3 to $28. Five million land mines have been produced in the United States since 1970. On January 12, 1995, thirty UN agencies and international nongovernmental organizations met to begin lobbying efforts to ban land mines. The effort is spearheaded by Physicians for Human Rights (PHR) and Handicap International (based in France). In late 1993 PHR published a 510-page book on land mines. Also see the *New York Times* (October 8, 1995, 3) and the *New York Times Magazine* (January 23, 1994).

6. According to Wang Xingjuan, president of the Women's Research Institute at the independent Chinese Academy of Management Science (*Wall Street Journal,* December 30, 1993). The legislation, the Maternal and Infantile

Health Care Law, went into effect in June 1995. It requires abortions of fetuses that have hereditary disease and restricts marriage of people with mental disabilities. I do not know if or how the disability rights groups in the PRC reacted to this. It should be noted that one of Deng Ziaoping's sons, Deng Fubang, heads the national organization of people with disabilities. Deng is a quadriplegic from a spinal cord injury he sustained during the Cultural Revolution.

7. In the Kallar community in Madurai, southern India, it became known that newborn girls were often fed poison berries to escape the ruinous effects of dowry. Of 640 families questioned, 51 percent admitted to killing a girl baby within a week of birth. Villagers were reported as defending the custom: "better to snuff a life at birth than to suffer lifelong misery." The conditions that give rise to this practice have implications for babies with disabilities. See "The Unwanted Sex," *New Internationalist* (February 1993).

8. This practice is not as common today as it once was, according to Dr. G. Ramadas, director of the All India Institute of Physical Medicine and Rehabilitation in Bombay.

9. People with disabilities in the United States have made important political advances in the last ten years. A progression of disability-related laws have been passed during this period which extend civil rights protection to people with disabilities in the areas of education (Individuals with Disabilities Education Act); housing (Fair Housing Amendments Act); and employment, transportation, and public access (Americans with Disabilities Act).

10. Lenin argued that this position was Marx's great economic insight: "Where the bourgeois economists saw a relation of things (the exchange of one commodity for another) Marx revealed a relation between people" ([1919] 1967b:209). Marx's comments are also useful here: "A negroe is a negroe. Only in certain conditions does he become a slave. A cotton-spinning machine is a machine for spinning cotton. Only under certain conditions does it become capital. Torn away from these conditions, it is as little capital as gold by itself is money, or sugar is the price of sugar" ([1849] 1961:28).

11. Meszaros extends his definition numerous times in the course of *Beyond Capital*. For instance, he calls it "the objectification of alien labor" (p. 809) and "the most comprehensively alienated mode of control in history, with its self-enclosed command structure" (p. 806).

12. It regulates this exchange on the basis of the amount of socially useful labor value that has gone into producing and distributing these commodities.

13. Exchange value implies something someone recognizes as having a worth to them which satisfies a need. Exchange value represents a market relation; it has a market value.

14. See *Mouth* 1995.

15. The *Mouth* takes its numbers from the *HCFA Financial Report* (FY 1994), *Facts and Trends* (1995), and Marion Merrell Dow's *Institutional Digest* (1995).

16. David Harvey's elegant *The Condition of Postmodernity* examines shifts in culture, economics, and time/space. Two excerpts are particularly relevant to my point. On the economic side: "Even though present conditions are very different in many respects, it is not hard to see how the invariant elements and

relations that Marx defined as fundamental to any capitalist mode of production still shine through, and in many instances with an even greater luminosity than before, all the surface froth and evanescence so characteristic of flexible accumulation" (pp. 187–188). On the ideological side: "But as Simmel (1978) long ago suggested, it is also at such times of fragmentation and economic insecurity that the desire for stable values leads to a heightened emphasis upon the authority of basic institutions—the family, religion, the state" (p. 171).

Chapter 4:   Culture(s) and Belief Systems

1. For a discussion of the Hubeer, see Helander 1995:73–93.

2. Paternalism has played a crucial role in the way in which societies and cultures have constructed the category "sick role." In *The Social System,* Talcott Parsons developed typologies that attempted to simplify the social roles different social strata played. One definition of encompassed people who met the "sick role" is as follows: not responsible for their sickness; exempted from typical tasks and responsibilities; and seek professional (usually medical) help.

3. The medicalization of disability has been treated at great length elsewhere (see, e.g., Fine and Asch 1988:40 n. 1; Shapiro 1993; Longmore 1987; Oliver 1990).

4. This is the case in the futuristic, cyberpunk novels of William Gibson (e.g., *Mona Lisa Overdrive*) and movies like Kathryn Bigelow's *Strange Days.*

5. These healers have a very interesting social role and relate differently to people with different disabilities. According to Asuni, "the care and treatment of persons with mental illness by the traditional healers [in Nigeria] generally involves the active participation of relatives of the mentally ill. In fact the relatives have to live with their ill member in the compound of the traditional healers to provide creature needs of the patient and also to participate in the healing rituals. The treatment consists of administration of herbs and performance of rituals with recitation of incantations" (1990:35–36).

6. I use "karma" in the popularly understood manner as destiny, although it more accurately means only activity.

7. No matter how conservative or eclectic the doctrine, language is recognized as crucially important to ideas and behavior. Jacques Lacan gave particular attention to the study of language because he knew speech was the medium for the psychoanalysis he practiced. Saussure's groundbreaking linguistics in the early twentieth century suggested that every word is stamped with the traces of how that language had been spoken before the words had actually been uttered. Because meaning is already determined *within language,* it is extraordinarily difficult to use a word in a new way. Even the most notorious opponents of causality acknowledge the impact of language. Bronislaw Malinowski, one of anthropology's early giants, who did not believe language contained any "theory" and who divided expression and behavior, paid great attention to language. Language is for Malinowski "a conditioning stimulus of human action and . . . becomes, as it were, a grip on things outside the reach of the speaker but within that of the hearers" ([1935]1964:59).

Chapter 5:   Consciousness and Alienation

1. For Marx, the estrangement of the worker from his work, especially the product of his work, is at the core of alienation. Alienation, in turn, masks the exploitation the worker is subjected to because the worker believes what he makes is legitimately owned by someone else (the owner, industrialist, investor, etc.). He does not realize he is not being paid for the product he makes but only for a small fraction of the product's worth. Profit is located in production, not in sales or marketing or the good looks of the boss, although all of these elements may influence the market. As profits are located in production (production is socially defined), so is exploitation. Exploitation is an economic relationship.

2. Braverman (1974) has been criticized for emphasizing the passive behavior of workers in the light of these evolving managerial strategies and not the role of resistance to these changes in the workplace. Also see Gordon, Edwards, and Reich 1982.

3. The diaspora of Palestinians is dramatic: 2 million live in the West Bank, Gaza, and the Golan Heights; another 3 million live in exile.

4. The important distinction is deaf culture, which, while quite controversial inside and outside the DRM, has a real history (in some parts of the world).

5. For a comprehensive bibliography on disability-related culture that includes literature, poetry, theater, and history, see Brown 1995.

Chapter 6:   Observations on Everyday Life

1. For example, although they are relatively numerous in Washington, D.C., and Minneapolis, sign language interpreters are not available in many parts of the United States. Many states do not subsidize personal assistance services; others pay up to $12 an hour (most pay minimum wage).

2. According to the UN, there are 70,000 amputees in Angola, 36,000 in Kampuchea, and 200,000 in Vietnam. See *In Motion* magazine, "Reaping a Grim Crop" (August 1995).

3. There was a documentary made about head injury and Golfus that was released in 1994 to critical acclaim: *When Billy Broke His Head and Other Tales of Wonder* (produced by Billy Golfus and David Simpson, Independent Television Services, St. Paul, Minn.).

4. Gladys Baez was one of the women memorialized in Margaret Randall's *Sandino's Daughters*.

5. Townships should not be equated with slums, although they are extremely poor. They more closely approximate cities in terms of their sheer size. There are many throughout South Africa.

6. Third World urban violence has been the subject of a great many books and films. I recommend the highly acclaimed Brazilian film *Pixote,* a violent story of how street kids survive in the urban environment (directed by Hector Babenco for NewYorker, 1981).

7. This assessment supports Marx's widely criticized assessment of the relationship between economic development and ideology: "In the social

production of their life, men enter into definite relations that are indispensable and independent of their will, relations of production which corresponds to a definite stage of development of their productive forces. The sum total of these relations of production constitutes the economic structure of society, the real foundation on which rises a legal and political superstructure and to which correspond definite forms of social consciousness" (Marx [1859] 1964b:11–12).

Chapter 7:   Empowered Consciousness and the Philosophy of Empowerment

1. For example, in perhaps the most important text on the subject, *History and Class Consciousness*, Georg Lukács never successfully shows *why* people move from false consciousness to "class consciousness." Lukács's brilliance is in his exposition of false consciousness through a series of exploratory vignettes. Lukács believes people have the innate capacity to move from reified (false) consciousness to revolutionary, class consciousness. He does not, however, describe how or why this happens for a few and not for most.

2. Whenever and wherever this transformation occurs, it produces recognition of the self on both the personal and the political levels. This transformation has been particularly important to feminist and multicultural studies. See Taylor 1994.

3. An argument advanced by the DRM's leadership is that employing people with disabilities is good for everybody. People with jobs pay taxes, contribute to society, get off the dole. This obligatory logic is never called into question. The possibility of full employment in a capitalist economy is no longer even considered viable in orthodox economic theory. Yet liberals within the DRM promote this pipe dream because they accept that capitalism works well and the reason for unemployment of people with disabilities is discrimination in the personnel office, the college admissions office, and so on. Many economists far removed ideologically from the left have demonstrated that unemployment is a necessary feature of capitalism because it is a drag on wages. The lower the wage, the higher the profit. Capital today not only requires relatively high levels of unemployment, it incessantly demands greater "wage flexibility" on the part of workers.

4. Tuk-tuks are prominent taxilike contraptions throughout Asia. They are often motorcycles with wooden frames to accommodate passengers. Peseros are minivans named for their once-upon-a-time fare, one peso.

Chapter 8:   The Organization of Empowerment

1. It took a monthlong sit-in and office takeover at the U.S. Department of Health, Education, and Welfare to force the secretary of HEW, Joseph Califano, to mandate its enforcement. There are a number of interesting accounts of this action. For example:

More than 150 people took over the federal building and remained for twenty-eight days. Ed Roberts left his new office as Director of the California Department of Rehabilitation to join the protest. Judy Heumann crossed the Bay from Berkeley to become one of the leaders of the takeover. Early in action, Heumann, in a statement reminiscent of freedom fighters of all ages, declared that "we will no longer allow the government to oppress disabled individuals. . . . We will accept no more discussion of segregation." . . . The Black Panthers and the Gray Panthers brought in food donated by Safeway and assisted with personal care needs. The siege remains the longest takeover of a federal building by any group in American history. (Brown 1995:57–58)

2. Driedger 1989 is a good history of the split and the subsequent formation of DPI (see esp. pp. 28–57).

3. Rehabilitation International (RI) remains much larger and more influential than DPI. In recent years, RI has added persons with disabilities to its executive committee, but it is still dominated by rehabilitation "professionals" (doctors, therapists, social workers, psychologists, etc.). Since the split, a number of disability rights activists have worked with both RI and DPI. RI is headquartered in New York City.

4. This was done with the assistance of Disabled International Support Effort, Ralf Hotchkiss, and others from the San Francisco Bay area.

5. CILs are not the only kinds of LAPCs. There are hundreds, probably thousands, of others. Often, disability rights activists question how authentic these organizations are and who controls them. An example of an authentic LAPC is the Hong Kong Federation of Handicapped Youth (HKFHY). The HKFHY not only provides self-help counseling and employment training, it has been very active in transportation advocacy throughout the colony. Leo Lam, the chairman of HKFHY's executive committee, is one of Hong Kong's leading disability rights advocates.

6. For an excellent example, see NACLA 1995, which covers Brazil's Movimiento dos Trabalhadores Rurais Sem Terra (Movement of Landless Rural Workers).

Chapter 9:   The Dialectics of Oppression and Empowerment

1. This is not to argue that poststructuralists/postmodernists do not see oppression. They do. And they would argue that their theories allow for resistance based on a politics of difference. I believe this is wishful thinking. If everyday life is *essentially* fragmented, the notions of oppression and justice are either effaced or atomized into oblivion. Of course, there is a range among these academics—from Iris Young to Jane Flax. Young, to her credit, has developed a space for justice within her fragmented world, something Michel Foucault also tried to do. Ironically, Foucault, contrary to many he influenced, problematized the omission of structures from analysis and action. Both the brilliance and the problems of Foucault's poststructuralism are shown in his studies of insanity and asylums, *Madness and Civilization* and *The Birth of the Clinic*. Foucault contends that people who are mentally ill are oppressed. He goes on at great length to show, however, that this oppression is site-specific, in this case, institutionally based in asylums and mental health clinics.

2. In its attack on the difference-blind concept of integration (Marable's inclusion tendency), the "politics of difference" unhesitatingly advocates that "social policy should sometimes accord special treatment to groups" (Young 1990: 158). The disability experience itself should caution the proponents of this view. Whereas it is easy to agree with Young that affirmative action, bilingual programs, and birthing rights for workers must be supported, it is similarly necessary to point out that people with disabilities have had more experience with "special treatment" than any other oppressed group. People with disabilities have been the "beneficiaries" of special programs for the last twenty years in the areas of employment, education, housing, transportation, and recreation. In all these instances, "special" has meant segregated and inferior. The DRM itself provides a critical response to the politics of difference. The DRM, in both the center and the periphery, has attempted two things simultaneously: it has demanded equality and inclusion while cultivating a growing sense of disability-based consciousness through peer counseling and self-help, community activities, and promotion of disability culture. The DRM, for the most part, has never tried to ignore the differences of people with disabilities. Where it is obvious that differences require appropriate consideration, the DRM has fought for the "reasonable accommodation" of people within the context of disability rights and integration. We are proud of our differences, but we know special treatment is inferior and feeds the ideology of inferiority as well.

3. Although Engels correctly links necessity with freedom, I believe freedom is more incremental. On Engels's notion of freedom, see Walicki 1995.

4. "Practical taxonomies, which are a transformed, misrecognizable form of the real divisions of the social order, contribute to the reproduction of that order by producing objectively orchestrated practices adjusted to those divisions" (Dirks, Eley, and Ortner 1994:159).

Bibliography

Abberley, P.
  1987.   "The Concept of Oppression and the Development of a Social
          Theory of Disability." *Disability, Handicap and Society* 2
          (1):5–19.
Ahmad, Aijaz.
  1992.   *In Theory.* London: Verso.
Albrecht, Gary L.
  1992.   *The Disability Business: Rehabilitation in America.* Newbury
          Park, Calif.: Sage.
Althusser, Louis.
  1964.   *For Marx.* London: Verso.
  1971.   *Lenin and Philosophy.* New York: Monthly Review Press.
Amin, Samir.
  1990.   *Maldevelopment: Anatomy of Global Failure.* London: Zed Press.
Amin, Samir, Giovanni Arrighi, Andre Gunder Frank, and Immanuel
  Wallerstein.
  1990.   *Transforming the Revolution: Social Movements in the World Sys-
          tem.* New York: Monthly Review Press.
Apple, Michael.
  1979.   *Ideology and Curriculum.* London: Routledge and Kegan Paul.
Apple, Michael, and Lois Weis
  1986.   *Ideology and Practice in Schooling.* Philadelphia: Temple Univer-
          sity Press.
Ashbar, Mark, ed.
  1994.   *Manufacturing Consent: Noam Chomsky and the Media.* Mon-
          treal: Black Rose Books.

Asuni, Tolani.
  1990.   "Nigeria: Report on the Care, Treatment and Rehabilitation of
           People with Mental Illness." *Views from Africa, India, Asia and
           Australia, Psychosocial Rehabilitation Journal* 49 (July):35–44.
Baldwin, James.
  1972.   *No Name in the Street.* New York: Doubleday.
Baran, Paul.
  1962.   *The Political Economy of Growth.* 2d ed. New York: Monthly Re-
           view Press.
Baran, Paul, and Eric Hobsbawm.
  1961.   "The Stages of Economic Growth." *Kyklos* 14, fasc. 2.
Bartky, Sandra Lee.
  1990.   *Femininity and Domination: Studies in the Phenomenology of
           Oppression.* New York: Routledge.
Beier, Ulli.
  1969.   "A Year of Sacred Festivals in One Small Yoruba Town." *Nigeria
           Magazine.*
Bell, Derrick.
  1992.   *Faces at the Bottom of the Well: The Permanence of Racism.* New
           York: Basic Books.
Bennets, L.
  1993.   "Letter from Las Vegas." *Vanity Fair* (September): 82–96.
Boggs, Carl.
  1984.   *The Two Revolutions: Gramsci and the Dilemmas of Western
           Marxism.* Boston: South End Press.
  1986.   *Social Movements and Political Power.* Philadelphia: Temple Uni-
           versity Press.
Bourdieu, Pierre, and Jean-Claude Passeron.
  1977.   *Reproduction in Education, Society, and Culture.* Trans. Richard
           Nice. London: Sage.
Bowles, Samuel, and Herbert Gintis.
  1976.   *Schooling in Capitalist America.* New York: Basic Books.
Bowman, Glenn.
  1994.   "A Country of Words: Conceiving the Palestinian Nation from
           the Position of Exile." In *The Making of Political Identities,* ed.
           Ernesto Laclau, 138–170. London: Verso.
Boylan, E. R.
  1991.   *Women and Disability.* London: Zed Books.
Braudel, Fernand.
  1979.   *The Structures of Everyday Life.* Vol.1 of *Civilization and Capi-
           talism, 15th–18th Century.* New York: Harper & Row.
Braverman, Harry.
  1974.   *Labor and Monopoly Capitalism: The Degradation of Work in the
           Twentieth Century.* New York: Monthly Review Press.
Brown, Steven E.
  1992.   "Creating a Disability Mythology." *International Journal of Re-
           habilitation Research* 15:227–233.

1995.   *Investigating Disability Culture: Final Report.* Washington, D.C.: National Institute on Disability Research and Rehabilitation.

Callahan, John.

1989.   *Don't Worry, He Won't Get Far on Foot: The Autobiography of a Dangerous Man.* New York: William Morrow.

1990.   *Do Not Disturb Any Further.* New York: William Morrow.

Callinicos, Alex.

1989.   *Against Postmodernism: A Marxist Critique.* Cambridge: Polity Press.

Camêra, Maria Luiza.

1981.   *Não Se Cria Filho Corm as Pernas.* Salvador, Brazil: Fundacão Cultural do Estado do Bahia.

Campbell, Joseph.

1988.   *The Power of Myth.* New York: Doubleday.

Canetti, Elias.

[1962] 1984.   *Crowds and Power.* New York: Farrar Straus and Giroux.

Carrillo, A. C., K. Corbett, and V. Lewis.

1982.   *No More Stares.* Berkeley: Disability Rights Education and Defense Fund.

Caws, Peter.

1994.   "Identity: Cultural, Transcultural, and Multicultural." In *Multiculturalism: A Critical Reader,* ed. David Theo Goldberg, 371–405. Cambridge, Mass.: Blackwell.

Charlton, James.

1992.   "Development and Disability: Voices from the Periphery." In *Traditional and Changing Views of Disability in Developing Societies,* 41–70. Monograph 53. Durban: University of New Hampshire, International Exchange of Experts and Information in Rehabilitation.

1994a.   "Religion and Disability." *Disability Rag* (Spring):17–25.

1994b.   "The Disability Rights Movement and the Left." *Monthly Review* 3 (46):77–85.

Chinweizu.

1987.   *The West and the Rest of Us: White Predators, Black Slaves and the African Elite.* Lagos, Nigeria: Pero Press.

Chomsky, Noam, and Edward S. Herman.

1988.   *Manufacturing Consent: The Political Economy of the Mass Media.* New York: Pantheon.

Cockcroft, James D., Andre Gunder Frank, and Dale L. Johnson.

1967.   *Capitalism and Underdevelopment in Latin America.* New York: Monthly Review Press.

Colby, Gerald, and Charlotte Dennett.

1995.   *Thy Will Be Done: The Conquest of the Amazon, Nelson Rockefeller and Evangelism in the Age of Oil.* New York: HarperCollins.

Cortazar, Julio.

[1966] 1987.   *Hopscotch.* Trans. Gregory Rabassa. New York: Pantheon Books.

Crewe, Nancy, and Irving Zola.
    1983.   *Independent Living for Physically Disabled People.* London:
            Jossey-Bass.
DeJong, Gerben.
    1979.   *The Movement for Independent Living: Origins, Ideology and Im-
            plications for Disability Research.* East Lansing: Michigan State
            University Press.
Deva, M. Parameshvara.
    1990.   "Psychosocial Rehabilitation in the Developing Worlds: Progress
            and Problems." In *Psychosocial Rehabilitation and Mental Illness:
            Views from Africa, India, Asia and Australia. Psychosocial Reha-
            bilitation Journal* 49 (July):21–34.
Dirks, Nicholas B., Geoff Eley, and Sherry B. Ortner, eds.
    1994.   *Culture/Power/History.* Princeton: Princeton University Press.
Dobb, Maurice.
    1946.   *Studies in the Development of Capitalism.* London: Oxford Press.
DPI Newsletter.
    1986.   Winnipeg: DPI.
Driedger, Diane.
    1989.   *The Last Civil Rights Movement: Disabled Peoples' International.*
            New York: St. Martin's Press.
Driedger, Diane, and Susan Gray, eds.
    1992.   *Imprinting Our Image: An International Anthology by Women
            with Disabilities.* Winnipeg: Gynergy Books.
Dunlap, Douglas A.
    1990.   "Rural Psychiatric Rehabilitation and the Interface of Community
            Development and Rehabilitation Services." In *Psychosocial Rehabil-
            itation and Mental Illness: Views from Africa, India, Asia and Aus-
            tralia. Psychosocial Rehabilitation Journal* 49 (July):67–90.
Eagleton, Terry, ed.
    1989.   *Raymond Williams: Critical Perspectives.* Boston: Northeastern
            University Press.
Edelman, Gerald M.
    1989.   *The Remembered Present: A Biological Theory of Consciousness.*
            New York: Basic Books.
Ellison, Ralph.
    [1947] 1989.   *Invisible Man.* New York: Vintage Books.
Engels, Friedrich.
    [1878] 1972.   *Anti-Duhring.* New York: International Publishers.
Eribon, Didier.
    1991.   *Michel Foucault.* Trans. Betsy Wing. Cambridge, Mass.: Harvard
            University Press.
Estrella, Aurora.
    1992.   "Philippine Experience in Promoting the Organization of Dis-
            abled Persons on a Self-Help Basis." In *Equalization of Opportu-
            nities,* 173–186. Bangkok: United Nations Economic and Devel-
            opment Commission for Asia and the Pacific.

Fanon, Frantz.
    1965.   *Studies in a Dying Colonialism.* Trans. Haakon Chevalier. New York: Monthly Review Press.
    1967.   *Black Skin, White Masks.* Trans. Charles Lam. New York: Grove Press.
    1968.   *The Wretched of the Earth.* Trans. Constance Farrington. New York: Grove Press.

Farber, B.
    1968.   *Mental Retardation: Its Social Context and Social Consequences.* Boston: Houghton Mifflin.

Ferguson, Ann.
    1989.   *Blood at the Root.* London: Pandora.

Fine, Michelle, and Adrienne Asch, eds.
    1988.   *Women with Disabilities: Essays in Psychology, Culture, and Politics.* Philadelphia: Temple University Press.

Finger, Anne.
    1993.   "Toward a Theory of Radical Disability Photography." *Disability Rag* (November):29–31.

Flax, Jane.
    1990.   *Thinking Fragments: Psychoanalysis, Feminism, and Postmodernism in the Contemporary West.* Berkeley: University of California Press.

Foucault, Michel.
    1965.   *Madness and Civilization: A History of Insanity in the Age of Reason.* Trans. Richard Howard. New York: Pantheon.
    1973.   *The Birth of the Clinic: An Archeology of Medical Perception.* Trans. A. M. Sheridan Smith. New York: Pantheon.
    1980.   *Power/Knowledge.* Ed. Colin Gordon. New York: Pantheon Books.

Frank, Andre G.
    1968.   *Capitalism and Underdevelopment.* New York: Monthly Review Press.
    1984.   *Critique and Anti-Critique.* London: Macmillan.

Frank, Gelya.
    1988.   "On Embodiment: A Case Study of Congenital Limb Deficiency in American Culture." In *Women and Disabilities: Essays in Psychology, Culture, and Politics,* ed. Michelle Fine and Adrienne Asch, 41–71. Philadelphia: Temple University Press.

Freire, Paulo.
    1968.   *Cultural Action for Freedom.* Cambridge, Mass.: Center for the Study of Change.
    1973.   *The Pedagogy of the Oppressed.* New York: Seabury Press.
    1987.   *Education for Critical Consciousness.* New York: Continuum.

Galeano, Eduardo.
    1985.   *Memory of Fire.* 3 vols. Trans. Cedric Belfrage. New York: Pantheon Books.

Gallagher, Hugh.
    1985.   *FDR's Splendid Deception.* New York: Dodd Mead.

Galler, Roberta.
1984.   "The Myth of the Perfect Body." In *Pleasure and Danger: Exploring Female Sexuality*, ed. Carole S. Vance, 165–172. Boston: Routledge & Kegan Paul.

Gamwell, Lynn, and Nancy Tomes.
1995.   *Madness in America: Cultural and Medical Perceptions of Mental Illness before 1914.* Ithaca: Cornell University Press.

Garza, Rolando.
1986.   "Socio-Economic and Cultural Problems Affecting the Delivery of Rehabilitation Services to Hispanic Blind and Visually Disabled Individuals." In *Equal to the Challenge: Perspectives, Problems and Strategies in the Rehabilitation of the Nonwhite Disabled*, ed. Sylvia Walker, Faye Belgrave, Alma Banner, and Robert Nichols, 67–70. Washington, D.C.: Howard University Bureau of Educational Research.

Gareffi, Gary, and Lynn Hempel.
1996.   "Latin America in the Global Economy: Running Faster to Stay in Place." In *Report on the Americas*, 18–27. New York: NACLA.

Gartner, Alan, and Dorothy Kerzner Lipsky.
1987.   "Beyond Special Education: Toward a Quality System for All Students." In *Harvard Educational Review* 57 (4):367–395.

Geertz, Clifford.
1973.   *The Interpretation of Cultures.* New York: Basic Books.

Genovese, Eugene D.
1976.   *Roll, Jordan, Roll: The World the Slaves Made.* New York: Vintage Books.

Gill, Carol.
1994.   "Questioning Continuum." In *The Ragged Edge: The Disability Experience from the Pages of the First Fifteen Years of the Disability Rag*, ed. Barrett Shaw, 44–45. Louisville: Avocado Press.

Girardin, Jean-Claude.
1972.   "Sartre's Contribution to Marxism." In *The Unknown Dimension: Western Marxism Since Lenin*, ed. Dick Howard and Karl E. Klare, 307–321. New York: Basic Books.

Giroux, Henry A.
1988.   *Ideology, Culture, and the Process of Schooling.* Philadelphia: Temple University Press.
1995.   "Insurgent Multiculturalism and the Promise of Pedagogy." In *Multiculturalism: A Critical Reader*, ed. David Theo Goldberg, 323–343. Cambridge, Mass.: Blackwell.

Goffman, Erving.
1963.   *Stigma: Notes on the Management of Spoiled Identity.* New York: Simon & Schuster.

Goldberg, David Theo, ed.
1994.   *Multiculturalism: A Critical Reader.* Cambridge, Mass.: Blackwell.

Golfus, Billy.
    1994. "The Do-gooder." In *The Ragged Edge: The Disability Experience from the Pages of the First Fifteen Years of the Disability Rag*, ed. Barrett Shaw, 165–168. Louisville: Avocado Press.
    1996. "A Church Wedding." *New Mobility* (December):41.
Gordimer, Nadine.
    1981. *July's People*. New York: Vintage.
Gordon, David M., Richard Edwards, and Michael Reich.
    1982. *Segmented Work, Divided Workers*. Cambridge: Cambridge University Press.
Gottlieb, Roger.
    1987. *History and Subjectivity: The Transformation of Marxist Theory*. Philadelphia: Temple University Press.
Gramsci, Antonio.
    [1931] 1974. *Prison Notebooks*. New York: International Publishers.
Granovetter, Mark S.
    1973. "The Strength of Weak Ties." *American Journal of Sociology* 78:1360–1380.
Grin, Patricia, Arthur M. Miller, and Gerald Grin.
    1980. "Stratum Identification and Consciousness." *Social Psychology Quarterly* 43:30–47.
Groce, Nora.
    1985. *Everyone Spoke Sign Language Here: Hereditary Deafness on Martha's Vineyard*. Cambridge, Mass.: Harvard University Press.
Groch, Sharon.
    1993. "Oppositional Consciousness: Its Manifestation and Development: A Case Study of People with Disabilities." Master's thesis, DePaul University.
Gutkind, Peter, and Immanuel Wallerstein, eds.
    1985. *The Political Economy of Contemporary Africa*. New York: Sage.
Habermas, Jürgen.
    1971. *Knowledge and Human Interests*. Boston: Beacon Press.
    1975. *Legitimation Crisis*. Boston: Beacon Press.
Hahn, Harlan.
    1988. "The Politics of Physical Difference: Disability and Discrimination." *Journal of Social Issues* 44:39–47.
    1989. "Disability and the Reproduction of Bodily Images: The Dynamics of Human Appearances." In *The Power of Geography: How Territory Shapes Social Life*, ed. J. Wolch and M. Dear. Boston: Homan.
Hall, Stuart.
    1991. "Ethnicity: Identity and Difference." *Radical America* 23, no. 4 (October/December):9–20.
Hartsock, Nancy.
    1983. *Money, Sex, and Power: Toward a Feminist Historical Materialism*. New York: Longman.

1990.   "Foucault on Power: A Theory for Women?" In *Feminism/Postmodernism*, ed. Linda J. Nicholson, 157–176. New York: Routledge.

Harvey, David.
1992.   *The Condition of Postmodernity.* Cambridge: Blackwell.

Hegel, G. W. F.
[1824] 1967.   *The Phenomenology of Mind.* New York: Harper & Row.

Helander, Bernhard.
1995.   "Disability as Incurable Illness: Health, Progress, and Personhood in Southern Somalia." In *Disability and Culture,* ed. Benedicte Ingstad and Susan Reynolds Whyte, 73–93. Berkeley: University of California Press.

Helander, Einar.
1993.   *Predudice and Dignity: An Introduction to Community-based Rehabilitation.* UN Development Program Report no. E93-III-B.3. New York: UNDP.

Helander, Einar, Padmani Mendis, Gunnel Nelson, and Ann Goerdt.
1993.   *Training the Disabled in the Community: A Manual on Community-based Rehabilitation for Developing Countries.* Geneva: WHO/UNICEF/ILO/UNESCO.

Henwood, Doug.
1996.   "The Free Flow of Money." In *Report on the Americas,* 11–17. New York: NACLA. January/February.

Hershey, Laura.
1995.   "False Advertising: Let's Stop Pity Campaigns for People with Disabilities." *Ms.* (March/April):96.

Hesperian Foundation.
1991.   "Newsletter from the Sierra Madre #25." Palo Alto, Calif.: Hesperian Foundation.

Hevey, David.
1992.   *The Creatures Time Forgot: Photography and Disability Imagery.* New York: Routledge.

Hobsbawm, E. J.
1975.   *The Age of Capital.* New York: Signet.
1995.   *The Age of Extremes.* New York: Vintage.

hooks, bell.
1990.   *Yearning: Race, Gender, and Cultural Politics.* Boston: South End Press.
1992.   *Black Looks: Race and Representation.* London: Turnaround.

Hurst, Rachel.
1995.   "Choice and Empowerment: Lessons from Europe." *Disability & Society* 10 (4):529–534.

IEEIR *Interchange.*
1993.   "Culture and Disability in the Pacific." University of New Hampshire, International Exchange of Experts and Information in Rehabilitation, Institute on Disability.

Ingstad, Benedicte, and Susan Reynolds Whyte, eds.
1995.   *Disability and Culture.* Berkeley: University of California Press.

International Center on Disability (ICD).
  1986.   "Bringing Disabled Americans into the Mainstream." ICD
           Survey of Disabled Americans. Conducted by Louis Harris
           and Associates for the International Center for the Disabled.
Jameson, Fredric.
  1986.   "Third World Literature in the Era of Multinational Capital."
           Social Text (Fall):65–88.
  1991.   *Postmodernism, or the Cultural Logic of Late Capitalism.* Durham,
           N.C.: Duke University Press.
  1996.   "Five Theses on Actually Existing Marxism." *Monthly Review.*
           (April):1–10.
Jonas, Suzanne.
  1991.   *Popular Movements: The Battle for Guatemala.* Boulder, Colo.:
           Westview Press.
Kailes, June.
  1992.   *Language Is More than a Trivial Concern.* Playa del Rey, Calif:
           Self-published.
Kristeva, Julia.
  1977.   *Powers of Horror: An Essay in Abjection.* New York: Columbia
           University Press.
Kroeber, A., and C. Kluckhorn.
  1952.   *Culture: A Critical Review of Concepts and Social Systems.* Cam-
           bridge, Mass.: Harvard University Press.
Kugelmass, Judy W.
  1989.   "The Indonesian System of Caring: Mental Handicap and
           Family Adaptation in West Java." In *Final Report to the
           International Exchange of Experts and Information in Re-
           habilitation.* Durban: University of New Hampshire, Institute
           on Disability.
Laclau, Ernesto, ed.
  1994.   *The Making of Political Identities.* London: Verso.
Laclau, Ernesto, and Chantel Mouffe.
  1985.   *Hegemony and Socialist Strategy: Towards a Radical Democratic
           Politics.* London: Verso.
Larana, Enrique, Hank Johnston, and Joseph R. Gusfield, eds.
  1994.   *New Social Movements: From Ideology to Identity.* Philadelphia:
           Temple University Press.
Leamon, Dick, and Yutta Fricke.
  1991.   *The Making of a Movement.* SAFOD Evaluation. Bulawayo, Zim-
           babwe: SAFOD.
Lenin, V. I.
  [1916] 1964. *Imperialism, the Highest Stage of Capitalism.* Vol. 22
                of *Collected Works.* Moscow: Progress Publishers.
  [1912] 1967a. *The Development of Capitalism in Russia.* Moscow:
                Progress Publishers.
  [1919] 1967b. *Marx-Engels-Marxism.* Moscow: Progress
                Publishers.

Lévi-Strauss, Claude.
  1963.   "The Structural Anthropology of Myth." Trans. Claire Jacobson
           and Brooke Schoepf. In *Structural Anthropology*. New York:
           Basic Books.
  1966.   *The Savage Mind*. Chicago: University of Chicago Press.
  [1955] 1992.   *Tristes Tropiques*. New York: Penguin Books.
Longmore, Paul K.
  1987.   "Screening Stereotypes: Images of Disabled People in Televi-
           sion and Motion Pictures." In *Images of the Disabled, Dis-
           abling Images*, ed. A. Gartner and T. Joe, 65–78. New
           York: Praeger.
Lorde, Audre.
  1984.   *Sister Outsider*. Trumansburg, N.Y.: Crossing Press.
Lukács, Georg.
  1971.   *History and Class Consciousness*. Trans. Rodney Livingstone.
           Cambridge, Mass.: MIT Press.
Lyotard, Jean-François.
  1984.   *The Postmodern Condition*. Minneapolis: University of Minnesota
           Press.
Maccahiwalla, P., and S. Warde, eds.
  1992.   "A Study of Prospects and Problems Faced by Paraplegics in
           Their Socioeconomic Rehabilitation." Bombay: The Paraplegic
           Foundation.
McLaren, Peter.
  1994.   "White Terror and Oppositional Agency: Towards a Critical Mul-
           ticulturalism." In *Multiculturalism: A Critical Reader*, ed. David
           Theo Goldberg, 45–74. Cambridge, Mass.: Blackwell.
Magubane, Bernard M.
  [1979] 1990.   *The Political Economy of Race and Class in South Africa*.
           New York: Monthly Review Press.
Mahfouz, Naguib.
  1991.   *Palace of Desire*. New York: Anchor Books.
Malinowski, Bronislaw.
  1954.   *Magic, Science and Religion*. Garden City, N.Y.: Doubleday An-
           chor.
  [1944] 1960.   *A Scientific Theory of Culture and Other Essays*. New York:
           Oxford University Press.
  [1935] 1964.   *Coral Gardens and Their Magic*. Bloomington: Indiana
           University Press.
Mallory, Bruce L.
  1992.   "Changing Beliefs about Disability in Developing Countries:
           Historical Factors and Sociocultural Variables." In *Tradi-
           tional and Changing Views of Disability in Developing Societies*.
           Monograph 53. Durban: University of New Hampshire,
           International Exchange of Experts and Information in
           Rehabilitation.

Mandel, Ernest.
  1962.   *Marxist Economic Theory.* New York: Monthly Review Press.
  1978.   *Late Capitalism.* Trans. Joris de Bres. London: Verso.
Marable, Manning.
  1995.   "History and Black Consciousness." In *In Defense of History: Marxism and the Postmodern Agenda. Monthly Review* (July/August).
Marcuse, Herbert.
  [1941] 1960.   *Reason and Revolution.* Boston: Beacon Press.
  1964.   *One-Dimensional Man.* Boston: Beacon Press.
Marx, Karl.
  [1849] 1961.   *Wage-Labor and Capital.* New York: International Publishers.
  [1867] 1964a.   *Capital.* New York: International Publishers.
  [1859] 1964b.   "Preface." In *A Contribution to the Critique of Political Economy.* Chicago: Kerr.
  [1857–1858] 1973.   *Grundrisse.* Trans. Martin Nicholaus. Middlesex: Peguin Books.
Marx, Karl, and Friedrich Engels.
  1936.   *Correspondence 1846–1895.* New York: International Publishers.
Masson, Jeffrey M.
  1988.   *Against Therapy.* Monroe, Maine: Common Courage Press.
Mayekiso, Mzwanelle.
  1995.   *Township Politics: Civic Struggles for a New South Africa.* New York: Monthly Review Press.
Mermelstein, David, ed.
  1976.   *Economics: Mainstream Readings and Radical Critiques.* 3d ed. New York: Random House.
Merleau-Ponty, Maurice.
  [1945] 1962.   *Phenomenology of Perception.* Trans. Colin Smith. London: Routledge & Kegan Paul.
  1968.   *The Visible and the Invisible.* Trans. Alphonso Lingis. Evanston: Northwestern University Press.
Meszaros, Istvan.
  1970.   *Marx's Theory of Alienation.* London: Harper Torchbooks/Merlin Press.
  1995.   *Beyond Capital.* New York: Monthly Review Press.
Mindes, Jerome.
  1991.   "A Study of Bilateral, Multilateral, and International Voluntary Efforts to Help China Rehabilitate People with Disabilities." Fellowship Report. IEEIR and World Rehabilitation Fund.
Mohanty, Chandra Talpade.
  1991.   "Introduction: Cartographics of Struggle: Third World Women and the Politics of Feminism." In *Third World Women and the Politics of Feminism,* ed. Chandra Talpade Mohanty, Ann Russo, and Lourdes Torres, 34–35. Bloomington: Indiana University Press.

Morrison, Toni.
    1970.   *The Bluest Eye*. New York: Washington Square Press.
    1993.   *Playing in the Dark: Whiteness and the Literary Imagination*.
             New York: Vintage.
Mouth.
    1995.   "What Would You Choose for this Child." Rochester, N.Y.: Free
             Hand Press.
Mukherjee, Ramkrishna.
    1955.   *The Rise of the East India Company*. Berlin: VEB Deutscher
             Verlag der Wissenschaften.
Murphy, Robert F.
    1987.   *The Body Silent*. New York: Henry Holt.
National Council on Disability (NCD).
    1991.   "Public Attitudes Toward People with Disabilities." Report.
             Louis Harris and Associates.
    1994.   "Persons with Disabilities Lag Behind Other Americans in
             Employment, Education, Income (Census Bureau Estimates
             There Are 49 Million Americans with Disabilities)." Washington,
             D.C.: National Organization on Disability.
National Council on the Handicapped (NCH).
    1983.   *National Policy for Persons with Disabilities*. Washington, D.C.
Nichols, Robert W.
    1992.   "An Examination of Some Traditional African Attitudes towards
             Disability." In *Traditional and Changing Views of Disability in
             Developing Societies*, 25–40. Monograph 53. Durban: University
             of New Hampshire, International Exchange of Experts and
             Information in Rehabilitation.
Nicholson, Linda J., ed.
    1990.   *Feminism/ Postmodernism*. New York: Routledge.
    1993.   "Ethnocentrism in Grand Theory." In *Radical Philosophy: Tradi-
             tion, Counter-Tradition, Politics*, ed. Roger S. Gottlieb, 48–64.
             Philadelphia: Temple University Press.
Nkrumah, Kwame.
    [1964] 1970.   *Consciencism: Philosophy and Ideology for Decolonization*.
                    New York: Monthly Review Press.
Noble, John H., Jr.
    1981.   *Population and Development Problems Relating to Disability Pre-
             vention and Rehabilitation*. New York: Rehabilitation Interna-
             tional.
North American Congress on Latin America (NACLA).
    1994.   "The Political Uses of Culture." In *Report on the Americas*. New
             York: NACLA. September/October, 15–43.
    1995.   "Brazil: The Persistence of Inequality." In *Report on the Ameri-
             cas*. New York: NACLA. May/June, 16.
O'Connor, James.
    1973.   *The Fiscal Crisis of the State*. New York: St. Martin's Press.
Oliver, Michael.
    1990.   *The Politics of Disablement*. New York: St. Martin's Press.

Oliver, Mike, and Gerry Zarb.
    1989.   "The Politics of Disability: A New Approach." *Disability, Handicap, & Society* 4 (3):219–240.

Ollman, Bertell.
    1971.   *Alienation.* New York: Cambridge University Press.
    1993.   *Dialectical Investigations.* New York: Routledge.

Parsons, Talcott.
    [1951] 1957.   *The Social System.* New York: Free Press.
    [1937] 1968.   *The Structure of Social Action.* 2 vols. New York: Free Press.

Polanyi, Karl.
    1944.   *The Great Transformation.* New York: Rinehart.

Poulantzas, Nicos.
    1975.   *Political Power and Social Classes.* New York: New Left Books.

Pryor, J.
    1989.   "When Breadwinners Fall Ill: Preliminary Findings from a Case Study in Bangladesh." *IDS Bulletin* 20(2): 49–57.

Randall, Margaret.
    1984.   *Sandino's Daughters.* Boston: South End Press.

Roberts, Edward V.
    1977.   "Foreword." In *Emerging Issues in Rehabilitation,* ed. S. S. Pflueger. Washington, D.C.: Institute for Research Utilization.

Romo, Alynne.
    1995.   "Black Rights in Latin America." *Heartland Journal* (Summer).

Rothenberg, Mel.
    1993–1994.   "Making Left Politics More than a Discourse." *Crossroads* (December/January).

Rousso, Harilyn.
    1988.   "Daughters with Disabilities: Defective Women or Minority Women?" In *Women and Disabilities: Essays in Psychology, Culture, and Politics,* ed. Michelle Fine and Adrienne Asch, 139–171. Philadelphia: Temple University Press.

Rowbotham, Sheila.
    1973.   *Women's Consciousness, Man's World.* New York: Penguin.

Russell, Marta.
    1994.   "Malcolm Teaches Us, Too." In *The Ragged Edge: The Disability Experience from the Pages of the First Fifteen Years of the Disability Rag,* ed. Barrett Shaw, 11–14. Louisville: Avocado Press.

Sahlins, Marshall.
    1976.   *Culture and Practical Reason.* Chicago: University of Chicago Press.

Said, Edward W.
    1993.   *Culture and Imperialism.* London: Chatto & Windus.

Sartre, Jean-Paul.
    [1943] 1957.   *Being and Nothingness: An Essay on Phenomenological Ontology.* Trans. Hazel E. Barnes. New York: Washington Square Press.

1968.   *Search for a Method*. Trans. Hazel E. Barnes. New York: Vintage
         Books.

1976.   *Critique of Dialectical Reason*. Trans. Hazel E. Barnes. New
         York: New Left Books.

Saussure, Ferdinand de.

[1915] 1966.   *Course in General Linguistics*. New York: McGraw-Hill.

Schilpp, Paul Arthur, ed.

1991.   *The Philosophy of Jean-Paul Sartre*. Lasalle, Ill.: Open Court.

Schmidt, James.

1985.   *Maurice Merleau-Ponty: Between Phenomenology and Structural-
         ism*. New York: St. Martin's Press.

Schneir, Miriam, ed.

1972.   *Feminism: The Essential Historical Writings*. New York:
         Vintage Books.

Shapiro, Joseph P.

1993.   *No Pity: People with Disabilities Forging a New Civil Rights Move-
         ment*. New York: Times Books.

Shaw, Barrett, ed.

1994.   *The Ragged Edge: The Disability Experience from the Pages of the
         First Fifteen Years of the Disability Rag*. Louisville: Avocado Press.

Smith, Adam.

1937.   *An Inquiry into the Nature and Causes of the Wealth of Nations*.
         New York: Random House.

Sontag, Susan.

1977.   *Illness as Metaphor*. New York: Farrar, Straus and Giroux.

1988.   *AIDS and Its Metaphors*. New York: Farrar, Straus and Giroux.

Southern Africa Federation of Disability (SAFOD).

1993.   *Disability Frontline*.

Soyinka, Wole.

1980.   *Ogun Abibmam*. Staffrider Series, no. 4. Johannesburg:
         Raven Press.

Stewart, Jean.

1989.   *The Body's Memory*. New York: St. Martin's Press.

Susman, Joan.

1993.   "Disability, Stigma and Deviance." In *Social Science Medicine*
         38:15–22.

Tanzer, Michael.

1995.   "Globalizing the Economy: The Influence of the IMF and World
         Bank." *Monthly Review* (September):1–15.

Taylor, George.

1994.   "The Politics of Recognition." In *Multiculturalism: A Critical
         Reader*, ed. David Theo Goldberg, 81–85. Cambridge, Mass.:
         Blackwell.

Thompson, E. P.

1963.   *The Making of the English Working Class*. New York: Vintage
         Books.

Thompson, John.
    1990.   *Ideology and Modern Culture*. Stanford: Stanford University Press.
Thomson, Rosemarie Garland.
    1995.   "Integrating Disability Studies into Existing Curricula: The Ex-
             ample of 'Women and Literature' at Howard University." Ed.
             Lennard J. Davis and Simi Linton. *Radical Teacher* 47:15–21.
Tropea, Joseph.
    1987.   "Bureaucratic Order and Special Children: Urban Schools
             1890s–1940s." *History of Education Quarterly* 27 (1):29–52.
Tucker, Bonnie P., ed.
    1994.   "Discrimination on the Basis of Disability: The Need for a Third
             Wave Movement." *Cornell Journal of Law and Public Policy* 2,
             no. 3 (Spring):253–264.
Turner, Brian.
    1984.   *The Body and Society*. Oxford: Basil Blackwell.
Turner, Terence.
    1995.   "Social Body and Embodied Subject: Bodiliness, Subjectivity, and
             Sociality among the Kayapo." *Cultural Anthropology* 10
             (2):143–170.
United Nations.
    1992.   *Human Rights and Disabled Persons*. Geneva: UN.
UNESCO.
    1995.   "Overcoming Obstacles to the Integration of Disabled People."
             London: Disability Awareness in Action.
UN International Labour Office (UNILO).
    1993.   "Listen to the People: A Guide for Planners of Disability Pro-
             grammes." Geneva: UNILO.
U.S. General Accounting Office.
    1991.   Report 216, February. Washington, D.C.
USDOE.
    1992.   *Disability Statistics Abstract*. Washington, D.C.: U.S. Department
             of Education, National Institute on Disability and Rehabilitation
             Research. May.
Volosinov, V. N.
    [1930] 1973.   *Marxism and the Philosophy of Language*. New York: Semi-
                    nar Press.
Wade, Cheryl Marie.
    1994.   "Disability Culture Rap." In *The Ragged Edge: The Disability Ex-
             perience from the Pages of the First Fifteen Years of the Disability
             Rag*, ed. Barrett Shaw, 15–18. Louisville: Avocado Press.
Walicki, Andrzej.
    1995.   *Marxism and the Leap to the Kingdom of Freedom*. Stanford: Stan-
             ford University Press.
Walker, Alice.
    1983.   *In Search of Our Mother's Gardens*. New York: Harcourt Brace
             Jovanovich.

Walker, Sylvia.
    1986.   "Attitudes toward the Disabled as Reflected in Social Mores in
                Africa." In *Childhood Disability in Developing Countries,* ed. Kofi
                Mofi, Sylvia Walker, and Bernard Charles, 239–249. New York:
                Praeger.
Wallerstein, Immanuel.
    1974.   *The Modern World System.* Vol. 1. New York: Academic Press.
    1986.   *Africa and the Modern World.* Trenton, N.J.: Africa World Press.
Werner, David.
    1979.   *Disabled Village Children: A Guide for Community Health Work-
                ers, Rehabilitation Workers, and Families.* Palo Alto, Calif.: Hes-
                perian Foundation.
West, Cornel.
    1993.   *Race Matters.* Boston: Beacon Press.
Williams, Eugene.
    1989.   "Surviving Without a Safety Net in Brazil." In *Ideas Study Visit
                Report.* International Exchange of Experts and Information in
                Rehabilitation. Oakland, Calif. WID.
Williams, Raymond.
    1973.   "Base and Superstructure." *New Left Review,* no. 82 (Novem-
                ber/December):3–16.
Wolf, Naomi.
    1991.   *The Beauty Myth: How Images of Beauty Are Used Against Women.*
                New York: William Morrow.
Wood, Ellen Meiksins.
    1986.   *The Retreat from Class: A New "True" Socialism.* London: Verso.
World Bank.
    1994.   *World Development Report 1994: Infrastructure for Development.*
                Oxford: Oxford University Press.
World Institute on Disability (WID).
    1995.   *Changing Lives.* Oakland, Calif.: WID.
Young, Iris Marion.
    1990.   *Justice and the Politics of Difference.* Princeton: Princeton Univer-
                sity Press.
Zahar, Renate.
    1974.   *Frantz Fanon: Colonialism and Alienation.* New York: Monthly
                Review Press.
Zizek, Slavoj, ed.
    1994.   *Mapping Ideology.* London: Verso.
Zola, Irving.
    1981.   *Missing Pieces: A Chronicle of Living with a Disability.* Philadel-
                phia: Temple University Press.
    1983.   "Toward Independent Living Living: Goals and Dilemmas." In
                Independent Living for Physically Disabled People, 344–356.
    1984.   "Does It Matter What You Call Us?" *Disability Quarterly* 4:1–2.
    1987.   "The Politicization of the Self-Help Movement." *Social Policy* 18
                (Fall):32–33.

Index

Designer: U.C. Press Staff
Compositor: BookMasters, Inc.
Text: 10/13 Galliard
Display: Galliard
Printer & Binder: BookCrafters